New Directions
in Public Health Care:
A Prescription for
the 1980s

NEW DIRECTIONS IN PUBLIC HEALTH CARE

A Prescription for the 1980s

THIRD EDITION

Cotton M. Lindsay, *Editor*

Alain Enthoven
W. Philip Gramm
Leon R. Kass
Keith B. Leffler
Jack A. Meyer
Charles E. Phelps
Thomas C. Schelling
Harry Schwartz
Arthur Seldon
David A. Stockman
Lewis Thomas

Transaction Books
New Brunswick (U.S.A.) and London (U.K.)

CONTENTS

vi

CONTRIBUTORS

ALAIN ENTHOVEN
Marriner S. Eccles Professor of Public and Private Management,
Professor of Health Care Economics, Stanford University

W. PIIILIP GRAMM
U.S. Congressman, 6th District, Texas

LEON R. KASS
Henry R. Luce Professor in the College,
The University of Chicago

KEITH R. LEFFLER
Assistant Professor of Economics, University of Washington

COTTON M. LINDSAY
Associate Professor of Economics, UCLA, Director, EAGLE Institute,
School of Business Administration, and Visiting Professor,
Emory University, Atlanta

JACK A. MEYER
Director of Special Projects, American Enterprise Institute

CHARLES E. PHELPS
Director, Regulatory Policies and Institutions Program,
Senior Staff Economist, The Rand Corporation

THOMAS C. SCHELLING
Lucius N. Littauer Professor of Political Economy,
John F. Kennedy School of Government, Harvard University

HARRY SCHWARTZ
Writer in Residence, Department of Surgery,
College of Physicians and Surgeons, Columbia University

ARTHUR SELDON
Editorial Director, The Institute of Economic Affairs, London

DAVID A. STOCKMAN
U.S. Congressman, 4th District, Michigan

LEWIS THOMAS
President and Chief Executive Officer,
Memorial Sloan-Kettering Cancer Center

EDITOR'S NOTE

Although the structure of this third edition is the same as the first two, several new chapters have been added to address current problems. Examining new evidence on Canada and Great Britain, I have written a new chapter with Arthur Seldon and supplied an entirely new chapter on the market for medical care. W. Philip Gramm and David Stockman analyze the problem of regulation and hospital costs as embodied in the administration's recent hospital cost containment proposal. Jack Meyer analyzes the three general classes of legislation dealing with national health insurance now before Congress. And Alain Enthoven presents his proposal for increased competition in the health care industry, examines the politics influencing the debate, and sketches scenarios for solution.

These chapters replace others in the first editions. In addition, Charles E. Phelps has revised and updated his earlier chapter on "Public Sector Medicine," and we are reprinting a short article by Dr. Lewis Thomas, President and Chief Executive Officer of Memorial Sloan-Kettering Cancer Center, as a concluding comment on the tenuous relation between health and health care. Original chapters by Leon Kass, Thomas Schelling, Arthur Seldon, and Keith Leffler/Cotton Lindsay are reprinted without change because they have not become dated by recent events.

Cotton M. Lindsay
Editor

Atlanta, Georgia
February 1980

PREFACE

Since the institute published the first two editions of this book in 1976, the public debate on national health insurance (NHI) has undergone several important changes. First, stringency on public budgets maintained high public concern about the costs of a full NHI program. Cost estimates of Medicare and Medicaid had greatly underestimated what became an enormous drain on public budgets, and rising public consciousness about costs has greatly intensified with the tax revolt of the past two years.

As budget limitations reduced prospects for a full, comprehensive plan, the policy debate broadened. The Carter administration began to emphasize its program for hospital cost containment, focusing on that medical sector which had shown greatest cost increases. Moreover, other proposals began to make their way through congressional committees to change in a fundamental way the incentives governing medical markets.

These new approaches—which seek, fundamentally, to increase competition among providers of medical care—have appeared at a time when it is becoming clear that more conventional regulatory efforts at cost control have not been successful in other countries, such as West Germany.

To address the new policy context, the institute asked Cotton M. Lindsay, editor of the first two editions, if he would oversee creation of a third—using what remained pertinent and commissioning new work to reflect changed circumstances.

We hope that this new edition will be valuable in clarifying issues in the public debate on this important subject.

> H. Monroe Browne
> President
> Institute for Contemporary Studies

San Francisco, California
February 1980

xi

HARRY SCHWARTZ

Introduction

The public debate on national health insurance. The Nixon,
Ford, and Carter proposals. Facts and assumptions in the current discussion—public health, access to care, the reasons
behind increased costs. "Powell's Law." The need for fresh
ideas.

The demand for the first two editions of this book was sufficiently strong to justify publication of the present revised third
edition within a relatively short time after the appearance of the
first. Such a demand is only one of many pieces of evidence of
the general interest in the American medical system and the importance of the current national debate on the subject. The
central issue of that debate is national health insurance. As this
is written there are numerous national health insurance bills
before Congress, most notably bills sponsored by President
Carter and by Senator Edward Kennedy, respectively. The

1

differences between the Carter and the Kennedy proposals figure prominently in the competition between the two men for the Democratic Party's presidential nomination in 1980. Despite the prominence of these candidates in the national debate, however, these two bills represent only a small portion of the spectrum of opinion in this field. In the center of that spectrum are those who suggest that only catastrophic insurance is needed since most Americans can afford the cost of routine medical care and minor illnesses. At one extreme of this spectrum are those who think the existing degree of government involvement in health care is excessive and who would cut back or eliminate entirely this involvement. At the other extreme are the supporters of the Dellums bill, sponsored by the California congressman, which would nationalize and socialize the American health care system, turning that system's personnel into hired government workers and establishing government ownership of all hospitals and other health care institutions.

It is notable that Republicans as well as Democrats have played significant roles in pushing for greater involvement of government in medicine. In early 1971 President Nixon came out for national health insurance and the following year he signed into law the Social Security Amendments of 1972 which significantly increased the scope of government-financed health care as well as of other governmental intrusions into the health system. During President Ford's brief tenure one of his earliest moves was to call for enactment of national health insurance, and before he left the White House he signed into law the health planning legislation which makes American medicine a competitor with American agriculture for the title of the most regulated and "planned" (in the Soviet sense of planning) section of the American economy.

This quasi-consensus at the highest levels of both American political parties reflects a number of shared assumptions as well as a common desire for political advantage. The shared assumptions are at least approximated by the "Findings" given at the beginning of the Carter national health insurance bill introduced in the fall of 1979. These contain the following assertions:*

The current health care system in the US is costly and inefficient, and does not provide needed health services to all Americans, millions of Americans lack insurance coverage for basic health services and protection against the rising cost of major illness,

as a result, the national health is seriously and adversely affected and this in turn seriously affects the general welfare,

to protect national health and, consequently, the general welfare, it is necessary to assure that adequate health care for all Americans is available and affordable.

The purposes of the Carter bill, as spelled out in its section 3, also throw light on widely shared assumptions. The bill's purposes are said to include improving "the quality of health care provided to Americans, and especially to the poor, to mothers, and to children, by increasing the availability and continuity of care and by emphasizing preventive health measures." Additionally it seeks to "reduce inflation in the health care industry by reducing unnecessary health care spending while providing fair compensation to those who furnish health care." The bill also seeks to "assure that all Americans have freedom of choice in their selection of physicians and other providers of health care (unless an individual voluntarily agrees to limit his choice of providers by enrolling in certain kinds of health care plans)." There is also talk of effecting savings from increased efficiency, encouraging "competition in the health care system through the growth of prepaid arrangements and other measures to stimulate greater efficiency and cost consciousness," and to "provide for health systems reform, especially with regard to the reduction of excess capacity in hospitals, and enhance federal efforts to develop needed health resources."

This summary of what might be called the conventional wisdom about the American health care system as of the end of the 1970s clearly implies that the health of the American people

---

*Material here is taken verbatim from the official HEW summary of the Carter "National Health Plan Act."

is unsatisfactory, that many Americans are denied medical care for economic reasons, and that the medical system is excessively costly and inefficient and must be radically restructured to give the desired health care to all Americans at satisfactory cost.

As is so often true, however, the conventional wisdom is open to sharp challenge. A heretical view would declare that this quasi-consensus has its facts wrong in part, and in part simply does not understand the real issue. It seems useful here to outline briefly the weaknesses of the dominant current of opinion on health care issues.

First, there is the matter of the health of the American people. Despite the usual rhetoric, official data show clearly that by all the most frequently used indices the health of the American people in the 1970s has been better than ever before, with the improvement continuing throughout the decade. The infant mortality rate in this country has plunged downward dramatically; by 1979 it was roughly half that of 1965. Similarly, the crude death rate of the United States set new lows in the mid- and late 1970s. And if one corrects the crude death rate to take account of the progressive aging of the American population, the decline in the death rate since World War II has been precipitous. Many of the current problems of American health care are in fact the price of success. More people than ever before are living into their seventies and eighties and even nineties, creating unprecedented needs for the care of additional millions of elderly people who are prone to suffer from the degenerative diseases of old age and whose treatment is difficult, expensive, and very often only palliative rather than curative. The increased number of elderly people now in the population is, of course, one reason for the climb in health care costs since the average person over sixty or seventy years of age needs far more medical and hospital services than does the average younger person.

Second, the complaints about access to medical care in the material quoted above seem to imply that large numbers of Americans simply have no possibility of seeing a doctor or of being hospitalized if required. Yet it is already a decade and a half since Congress passed into law the Medicare and Medicaid legislation providing government-financed medical care for persons sixty-five years old and over and for the poor. The statistics that have been gathered show clearly that in the present era there is no fixed direct relationship between, say, access to a physician and family income such as is implicitly assumed in the conventional rhetoric. Actually, low, middle, and upper income Americans in the 1970s have, on average, visited a physician roughly the same number of times on a per capita basis.

It may be argued that poverty is often the result of illness and that in some ideal, just society the poor would see doctors far more often than those above them in the income scale. But what is evident from the data is that the overwhelming majority of Americans have access to whatever physician and hospital services they need and do use them. It is perhaps a commentary on how stereotyped and mindless is the "lack of access" argument that many of those who mouth it complain simultaneously of excessive numbers of physicians and unneeded hospitals and hospital beds in this country. This rejoinder does not in any way deny that there are areas of the United States—particularly in rural regions—where there are at times no physicians or grossly inadequate numbers of physicians. But such areas are very much the exception and do not reflect in any way the situation in the areas where most Americans live. The inner-city slum districts which are often cited as regions of gross doctor shortage are frequently the sites of major teaching hospitals which see tens of millions of hospital outpatients and emergency room visitors annually.

Third, on the issue of costs, it is astonishing how rarely it is pointed out that the rapid growth of health care costs in this country has resulted from the increasing separation between receipt of medical services and out-of-pocket payment for them. The majority of Americans today, for example, have hospital insurance either from Blue Cross, Blue Shield, or from a private

health insurer such as Prudential or Equitable, or from
Medicare, Medicaid, or some other government program. Given
the fact that most Americans don't pay the cost of hospital care
from their own pockets, it is little wonder that hospital costs
have shot up more rapidly than any others in the health care
field. In this situation neither patients nor doctors have any incentive to minimize the use or the cost of hospital care, while
both have every reason to demand "the best care." The latter is
usually defined in this country as care given with the latest
medical technology—CAT-scanners, cardiac and other intensive care units, kidney dialysis and transplantation facilities,
heart catheterization units, etc., etc. If health care is a human
right, as the true believers argue, then why should the individual
patient or doctor settle for anything but the best—which is also
usually the most costly. People who are economical about medical care, and who hesitate to see a doctor or to enter the hospital
when they have to pay out of their own pockets, frequently
adopt a far more permissive attitude when somebody else pays
for them either through employer-paid insurance premiums or
through tax-financed Medicare and Medicaid.

Finally there is the question of why so many advocate some
comprehensive system of national health insurance when it is
already clear that partial approaches to this goal, through both
private health insurance and through government-financed
Medicare and Medicaid, are responsible for the cost explosion in
American health care since 1965. Won't making all health care
for everybody seem "free" worsen the situation by still further
diminishing incentives toward economy in this field?

Unfortunately, this central question is rarely addressed can-
didly in public debate on the issue. To the extent it is faced,
assurances are given that cost constraints under national health
insurance will bring the financial load under control. But there
are already government and privately sponsored cost constraints in place and so far they show little impact. Millions of
dollars have been spent during this past decade on Professional
Standards Review Organizations (which limit hospital stays of

sick patients) and Health Systems Agencies (the local planning groups throughout the country), but the cost of medical care continues undeviatingly upward.

The reality that nobody in power wants to face is expressed by what I have called "Powell's Law"—after J. Enoch Powell, the controversial British conservative politician—which was formulated after Mr. Powell had spent several years in the early 1960s as the British cabinet member in charge of Britain's National Health Service. The law simply notes that the potential demand for "free" health care is infinite. If a patient is dying, there is always another specialist who might be called, another expensive test that might be conducted, etc., etc. And as for those with emotional problems and the retarded and autistic children and others similarly unfortunate, entire corps of experts could be used for each case—with unfortunately little guarantee of achieving what the relatives of these patients want so desperately: a complete and decisive cure that will make the afflicted person a normal, happy, contributing member of society.

The practical impact of Powell's Law is that every system of comprehensive national health insurance must inevitably and certainly become a scheme for rationing health care services, for helping some and denying others. This follows because no society, including our own, is willing to give more than a finite and limited amount of resources for health care. But finite resources cannot satisfy infinite demands.

The real situation has been suggested by the ambiguous adjectives in the material quoted above from the Carter bill. That bill speaks of "adequate" health care and "unnecessary" health care, but what do these terms mean? What can be "adequate" health care in a world where everyone must die, including those who provide health care? When Senator Kennedy's son had cancer, the senator assembled experts from all over the United States to consider his son's problem and to counsel on what should be done. Does Senator Kennedy intend that his bill give every cancer victim the same generous availability to world-famous consultants at no cost to him? When the late Senator Humphrey was in his last years of life with bladder cancer, he went to New York's Memorial Hospital for one operation and to the University of Minnesota's medical school for another operation as well as using the best government medical facilities available in Washington. Will the Carter bill assure every cancer sufferer the same access to the best care in the land? Of course not. It would be too expensive.

But reality is usually not realized before a nation has riveted the chains of a national health insurance system upon its people. It is only afterward that the real debate begins: Who should be denied the needed care? The old who are no longer productive? The kidney disease victims whose treatment by dialysis is so expensive? The smokers who have brought their lung cancer upon themselves? The autistic children whom nobody knows how to cure anyway? The infants born with *spina bifida* or other incapacitating birth defects? The list of such unfortunates is almost endless.

There are, of course, those who think this dilemma can be circumvented. Some offer the so-called Health Maintenance Organizations (HMOs) in which doctors are paid a fixed fee for each patient and thus encouraged to do as little as possible—subject to the malpractice laws and to the fact that patients can switch to other providers if they are sufficiently unhappy—so as to maximize their profits. Others see the saving grace in injecting a large element of competition into the medical marketplace, a marketplace they argue has been dominated by monopolistic and noncompetitive doctors. The holders of these views are entitled to express their opinions and to support their proposals, as some do in this volume. But ultimately the reader must ask whether these arrangements introduce fundamental changes or merely shift the obligation of rationing health care from Washington to those who make policy for HMOs and health insurance companies.

The issues in the field of health care, in short, are by no means simple, nor are the solutions offered of certain and guaranteed efficacy. This is a field which needs fresh thinking and new ideas to test both the conventional wisdom and its present chief alternatives.

This volume's chief merit is that it presents abundant material to help all who would participate seriously in this major and most important part of the national debate and dialogue.

1

LEON R. KASS

Medical Care and the Pursuit of Health*

Health, unhealth, and the objectives of medical science. Socrates on health and on the individual's responsibility. Seven rules for good health. The medical profession and the community. The aim of national health policies: economic equality.

American medicine is not well. Though it remains the most widely respected of professions, though it has never been more technically powerful, it is in trouble both from without and from within.

Symptoms and signs of the trouble abound. Medical care is very costly and not equitably available. The average

*Adapted and condensed from "Regarding the End of Medicine and the Pursuit of Health," *The Public Interest*, no. 40 (Summer 1975), pp. 11–42.

doctor sees many more patients than he should, yet many fewer than would like to be seen. On the one hand the physician's powers and prerogatives have grown as a result of new technologies yielding new modes of diagnosis and treatment and new ways to alter the workings of the body. His responsibilities have grown as well, partly due to rising patient and societal demands for medical help with behavioral and social problems. On the other hand, the physician's new powers have brought new dilemmas, concern over which has led to new attempts to regulate and control his practices. More and more doctors are being dragged before the bar, and medical malpractice insurance has become alarmingly scarce and exorbitantly expensive.

Health care has become an important political issue. A right to health is frequently claimed and embraced by politicians. Recent legislation has put the federal government most directly into the lifesaving business, obliging it to pay for kidney machines for anyone in need. Professional Standards Review Organizations are already on stage, various plans for national health insurance are waiting expectantly in the wings, and it is rumored that a national health service—i.e., socialized medicine—may soon receive an audition.

The most widely discussed remedies for the so-called "medical care crisis" address economic or organizational matters: more money for training more physicians and for more research, more money to cover costs of medical care, more planning to make more and better use of available resources. These proposals all tacitly endorse both the goals and the methods of modern medical practice: we are doing the right things so let's have more of the same—better hospitals, more sophisticated equipment, newer drugs—only let's spread the benefits more fairly, eliminate inefficiency in the "delivery" of care, and insure ourselves against the rising costs.

Yet it is not so clear that we really need more of the same. Before rushing to decide these admittedly important economic and administrative issues and before deciding to pour vast sums of federal money into health insurance, we ought to consider carefully and thoroughly some rather fundamental yet often neglected questions: What is the proper end of medicine and of our public health policy? What are the best means for achieving this end? Assuming that *health* is our goal, are we wise in relying so heavily on modern medicine whose focus is primarily *disease* and therapy?

One must, of course, recognize therapeutic medicine's *past* contributions to healthiness, most prominently in its victories against infectious diseases and vitamin and hormone deficiencies. But it is far from clear that we can expect comparable improvements in the future by pursuing the successful ways of the past. To what extent does or can the so-called health care delivery system deliver or foster improved health for the American people? How do we become and remain healthy?

The purpose of this essay is to promote discussion of some of these fundamental questions, thereby providing a broader perspective in which to consider the various issues regarding national health insurance.

WHAT IS "HEALTH"?

Before turning to the question of what we can do to become healthier, we need to delimit what we mean by "health." Our view of health needs to be protected against the twin dangers of expansion and contraction, both actively at work today. On the one hand there is the cosmic view of health in which health is conflated with self-contentment or happiness and with good behavior or virtue. This view gains theoretic support partly from the open-ended character of some contemporary notions of mental health and practical support from the growing requests by individuals and communities for doctors to lend their technical and manipulative skills to serve nontherapeutic ends (e.g., pills to enliven a dull evening or to quiet a restless schoolboy or psychosurgery to tame a repeatedly violent criminal). On the other hand there is the constricted—not to say absent—view of health that informs today's medical profession, which bends all its energies fighting this disease or that but gives little attention to overall healthiness.

The pursuit of health needs also to be distinguished from the pursuit of longevity. Thus, with some misgivings, I would suggest that the prolongation of life or the prevention of death cannot be a major goal of medicine or of our health policy. It is not so clear that this is a false goal, especially as it is so intimately connected with the medical art and so often acclaimed as the first goal of medicine or at least its most beneficial product. Yet *to-be-alive* and *to-be-healthy* are not the same, though the first is both a condition of the second and, up to a point, a consequence. But no matter how desirable life may be—and clearly to be alive *is* a good, and a condition of all the other human goods—for the moment let us notice that the prolongation of life is ultimately an impossible—or rather an unattainable—goal for medicine. For we are all born with those twin inherited and inescapable "diseases," aging and mortality. To be sure, we can still achieve further reductions in *premature* deaths; but it often seems doubtful from our words and deeds that we ever regard any particular death as other than premature, as a failure of today's medicine hopefully avoidable by tomorrow's.

If medicine aims at death prevention rather than at health, then the medical ideal ever more closely to be approximated must be bodily immortality. Strange as it may sound, this goal really *is* implied in the way we as a community evaluate medical progress and medical needs. We go after the diseases that are the leading causes of death rather than those that are the leading causes of ill health. We evaluate medical progress and compare medicine in different nations in terms of mortality statistics. We ignore the fact that we are merely changing one set of fatal illnesses or conditions for another, and not necessarily for a milder or more tolerable one. We rarely stop to consider of what and how we shall spend our last years once we can cure cancer, heart disease, and stroke.

I am not suggesting that we cease investigating the causes of these diseases. On the contrary, medicine *should* be interested in preventing these diseases or, failing that, in restoring their victims to as healthy a condition as possible. But it is primarily because they are causes of *unhealth*, and only secondarily because they are killers, that we should be interested in preventing or combating them. That their prevention and treatment may enable the prospective or actual victims to live longer may be deemed in many cases an added good, though we should not expect too much on this score. The complete eradication of heart disease, cancer, and stroke—currently the major mortal diseases—would, according to some calculations, extend the average life expectancy at birth only by approximately six or seven years and at age sixty-five by no more than a year and a half to two years.[1] Medicine's contribution to longer life has nearly reached its natural limit.

If health is different from happiness and virtue and more than mere life but less than incorruptibility, what then can it be? Is it a positive quality or condition or merely the absence of some negative quality or condition? Is one necessarily "healthy" if one is not ill or diseased? One might infer from modern medical practice that health is simply the absence of all known diseases. Harrison's textbook, *Principles of Internal Medicine,* is a compendium of diseases and, apart from the remedies for specific diseases, contains no discussion of regimens for gaining and keeping health. Indeed, health is never explicitly discussed and the term "health" does not even occur in the index.

Clinical medicine's emphasis on disease and its cure is readily understood. It is the sick and not the well who seek out medical advice. The doctor has long been concerned with restoration and remedy, not with promotion and maintenance, originally the responsibilities of gymnastic and dietetics. This orientation has been encouraged by the analytic and reductive approach of modern medical science and by the proliferation of known diseases and treatments—both leading to a highly specialized but highly fragmented medicine. Doctors are too busy fighting disease to be bothered much about health, and up to a point this makes sense.

Yet among pediatricians, with their well-baby clinics and their concern for normal growth and development, we can in fact see medicine clearly pointing *to* an overall good rather than *away* from particular evils. The same goal also informs the practices of gymnastic (physical fitness programs) and of dietetics. Together these examples provide a provisional ground for the view that health is a good in its own right, not merely a privation of one or all evils. Though we may be led to *think* about health and to discover its existence only through discovering and reflecting on *departures* from health, health would seem to be the primary notion. Moreover, disease, as the generic name for the cluster of symptoms and identifiable pathological conditions of the body, is not a notion symmetrical with or opposite to health. Health and *unhealth*—i.e., health and falling short of health—are contraries, not health and disease. For, as we know all too well, we may feel ill and function poorly in the complete absence of disease.

I have tried elsewhere to provide the beginnings of a positive notion of health—one which would avoid the cosmic dimensions of the World Health Organization's definition, "A state of complete physical, mental, and social well-being"—by emphasizing two related notions: wholeness and well-working (Kass 1975). Against the current reductionist and specialized views, I have argued that one must look to the workings of whole organism to discover its healthiness.

What, for example, is a healthy squirrel? Not a picture of a squirrel, not really or fully the sleeping squirrel, not even the aggregate of his normal blood pressure, serum calcium, total body zinc, normal digestion, fertility, and the like. Rather, the healthy squirrel is a bushy-tailed fellow who looks and acts like a squirrel; who leaps through the trees with great daring; who gathers, buries, and covers but later uncovers and recovers his acorns; who perches out on a limb cracking his nuts, sniffing the air for smells of danger, alert, cautious, with his tail beating rhythmically; who chatters and plays and courts and mates, and rears his young in large improbable-looking homes at the tops of trees; who fights with vigor and forages with cunning, who shows spiritedness, even anger, and more prudence than many human beings.

Although it will prove more difficult to describe in this way the healthy human being, it nevertheless seems reasonable to think of health as a natural norm, as a state of being that reveals itself in activity as a standard of bodily excellence or fitness relative to each species and to some extent to individuals, recognizable if not definable, and to some extent attainable. If one prefers a more simple formulation I would say that health is "the well-working of the organism as a whole," or again, "an activity of the living body in accordance with its specific excellences."

THE PURSUIT OF HEALTH

Having thus identified health as the goal of medicine and of our health policies, we turn next to consider how it might be better attained. Curiously, it will soon become apparent that medicine itself, understood as the treatment of disease, may contribute relatively little to our becoming and remaining healthy.

Though health is a natural norm and though nature provides us with powerful inborn means of preserving and maintaining a well-working wholeness, it is wrong to assume that health is the simply given and spontaneous condition of human beings and unhealth the result largely of accident or of external invasion. In the case of nonhuman animals, such a view could perhaps be defended. Animals instinctively eat the right foods (when available) and act in such a way as to maintain their naturally given state of health and vigor. Animals do not overeat, undersleep, knowingly ingest toxic substances, nor permit their bodies to fall into disuse through sloth, watching television and riding in automobiles, transacting business, or writing articles about health. For us human beings, however, even a healthy nature must be nurtured and maintained by effort and discipline if it is not to become soft and weak and prone to illness, and certain excesses and stresses must be avoided if this softness is not to spawn overt unhealth and disease. One should not, of course, underestimate the role of germs and other hostile agents working from without; but I strongly suspect that the germ theory of disease has been oversold and that the state of "host resistance," and in particular the immunity systems, will become increasingly prominent in our understanding of both health and disease.

Once the distinction is made between health nurture and maintenance on the one hand and disease prevention and treatment on the other, it becomes immediately clear that bodily health does not depend only on the body and its parts. It depends decisively on the psyche with which the body associates and cooperates. A few examples will make this clear if it is not already obvious. Some disorders of body are caused, at least in part, by primary problems of soul (psyche); the range goes from the transitory bodily effects of simple nervousness and tension headaches through the often severe somatic symptoms of depression (e.g., weight loss, insomnia, constipation, impotence) to ulcers and rheumatoid arthritis. Other diseases are due specifically to some aspect of the patient's way of life: cirrhosis in alcoholics, hepatitis in drug addicts, special lung diseases in coal miners, venereal disease in prostitutes.

But the dependence goes much farther than these clear psychosomatic and sociosomatic interactions. In a most far-reaching way our health is influenced by our temperament, our character, our habits, our whole way of life. This fact was once better appreciated than it is today.

In a very early discussion of this question in the Platonic dialogue *Charmides*, Socrates criticizes Greek physicians for foolishly neglecting the whole when attempting to heal a part. He argues that "just as one must not attempt to cure the eyes without the head or the head without the body, so neither the body without the soul." In fact, one must care "first and most" for the soul if one intends for the body to be healthy. If the soul is moderate and sensible it will not be difficult to effect health in the body; if not, health will be difficult to procure. Greek medicine fails, it is charged, because men try to be physicians of health and moderation separately from each other.

Socrates does not say that excellence of soul and excellence of body are one and the same; indeed, health is clearly distinguished from moderation. Rather, the claim is that health is at least in large part affected by or dependent upon virtue, that being well in body has much to do with living well, with good habits not only of body but of life.

Now Socrates certainly knew, perhaps better than we, that accident and fortune can bring harm and ill-health even to well-ordered bodies and souls. He knew about inborn diseases and seasonal maladies and wounds sustained in battle. He knew that health, though demanding care and discipline and requiring a certain control of our bodily desires, was no sure sign of virtue—and that moderation is not all of virtue. He knew too, as we know, human beings whose healthiness was the best thing about them, and he knew also that to be preoccupied with health is either a sign or a cause of a shrunken human life. Yet he also clearly knew what we today are altogether too willing to forget, that *we are in an important way responsible for our state of health*, that carelessness, gluttony, drunkenness, and sloth take some of their wages in illness. At a deeper level, he knew that there was a connection between the fact that the human soul aspires beyond mere self-preservation and the fact that men, unlike animals, can make themselves sick and feverish. He knew, therefore, that health in human beings depends not only on natural gifts but also on taming and moderating the welcome yet dangerous human desire to live better than sows and squirrels.

Today we are beginning again to consider that Socrates was possibly right, that our way of life is a major key to our sickness and our health. I would myself guess that well more than half the visits to doctors are occasioned by deviations from health for which the patient or his way of life are in some important way responsible. Most chronic lung diseases, much cardiovascular disease, most cirrhosis of the liver, many gastrointestinal disorders (from indigestion to ulcers), numerous muscular and skeletal complaints (from low back pain to flat feet), venereal disease, nutritional deficiencies, obesity and its consequences, and certain kinds of renal and skin infections are in important measure self-induced or self-caused—and contributed to by smoking, overeating, overdrinking, eating the wrong foods, inadequate rest and exercise, and poor hygiene. To these conditions must be added the results of trauma—including automobile accidents, in which drunkenness plays a leading part—and suicide attempts as well as accidental poisonings, drug abuse, and many burns. I leave out of the reckoning the as yet poorly studied contributions to unhealth of all varieties made by the special stresses of modern urban life.

There are even indications that cancer is in some measure a disease of how we live, even beyond the clear correlations of lung cancer with smoking and cancer of the cervix with sexual promiscuity and poor sexual hygiene. If the incidence of each kind of cancer could be reduced to the level at which it occurs in the population in which its incidence is lowest, there would be 90 percent less cancer. Recent studies show that cancers of all sorts—not only cancers clearly correlated with smoking and drinking—occur less frequently among the clean-living Mormons and Seventh Day Adventists.

The foregoing, it will be noted, speaks largely about disease and unhealth and about the role of our excesses and deficiencies in bringing them about. Unfortunately, we know less about what contributes to healthiness, as nearly all epidemiological studies have been studies of disease. But in the last few years there have appeared published reports of a most fascinating and important series of epidemiological studies on *health* conducted by Dean Lester Breslow and his colleagues at the UCLA School of Public Health. Having first developed a method for quantifying, albeit crudely, one's state of health and well-functioning, they investigated the effect of various health practices on physical health status. They have discovered, empirically, seven independent "rules" for good health which correlate very well with healthiness and also with longevity. People who follow all seven rules are healthier and live longer than those who follow six, six more than five, and so on, in perfect order. Let me report two of their more dramatic findings: The physical health status of those over seventy-five who followed all the "rules" was about the same as those aged thirty-five to forty-four who followed fewer than three, and a person who follows at least six of the seven rules has an eleven-year longer life expectancy at age forty-five than someone who has followed less than four. Moreover, these differences in health connected with health practices persisted at all economic levels and, except at the very lowest incomes, appeared largely independent of income (Belloc and Breslow 1972; Belloc 1973).

The seven "rules" are: (1) don't smoke cigarettes, (2) get seven hours of sleep, (3) eat breakfast, (4) keep your weight down, (5) drink moderately, (6) exercise daily, and (7) don't eat between meals. ("Visit your doctor" is not on the list, though I must confess that I cannot find out if this variable was investigated.) It seems that Socrates—and also Grandmother—may have been on the right track.

One feels, I must admit, a bit foolish in the latter half of the twentieth century, which boasts the cracking of the genetic code, kidney machines, and heart transplants, to be suggesting the quaint formula, "Eat right, exercise, and be moderate, for tomorrow you will be healthy." But quaint formulas need not have been proven false to be ignored, and we will look far more foolish if Breslow and his colleagues are onto something which, in our sophistication, we choose to overlook.

IMPLICATIONS FOR POLICY

What might all this point to for medicine and for public policy regarding health? Let me try to sketch out in outline some implications of the preceding sections which, as a point of departure, I would summarize in this way: Health and only health is the doctor's proper business; but health, understood as well-working wholeness, is not the business only of doctors. Health is, in different ways, everyone's business, and it is best pursued if everyone regards and minds his *own* business—each of us his own health, the doctor the health of his patient, public health officials and legislators the health of the citizens.

With respect to the medical profession itself, there is a clear need to articulate and delimit the physician's domain and responsibilities to protect against expansion and contraction. The more obvious and perhaps greater danger seems to be expansion, given the growing technological powers that can serve nontherapeutic ends and the rising demands to put these powers to nonmedical uses. The medical profession must take the initiative in establishing and policing the necessary boundaries. The American Medical Association, the state and county medical societies, and the various specialty organizations would do well to review current practices and anticipated new technologies in the light of this problem and to offer guidance to their members. In some cases they might well try to discourage or proscribe certain quasi-medical or extra-medical uses of medical technique. For example, the American College of Obstetrics and Gynecology should consider regulations barring its members from helping prospective parents to determine or select the sex of their child-to-be; or the Amercan Association of Neurological Surgeons could establish strict guidelines for the permissible uses, if any, of destructive brain surgery for the sake of modifying behavior.

But the biggest problem is how to protect the boundaries of the medical domain against unreasonable *external* demands for expansion. The movement towards consumer control of medicine, the call for doctors to provide "therapy" for social deviants and criminal offenders, and the increasing governmental regulation of medical practice all run the great risk of transforming the physician into a mere public servant, into a technician or helper for hire. Granted, the doctor must not be allowed to be a tyrant. But neither must he become a servant. Rather, he must remain as a leader and a teacher. The community must respect the fact that medicine is an art and that the doctor rightly is a man of expert knowledge deserving more than an equal voice in deciding what his business is. Though one may rightly suspect *some* of the motives behind medicine's fear of governmental intrusion, one must acknowledge the justice of at least this concern: once the definition of health care and the standards of medical practice are made by outsiders—and the national health insurance schemes all tend in this direction, at the very least, by determining what will be paid for—the physician becomes a mere technician.[2]

Yet if the medical profession wants to retain its rightful claim to set the limits of its role, it must not only improve its immunity against foreign invasions seeking to enlarge its domain but must also work to restore its own wholeness. The profession must again concern itself with health, with wholeness, with well-working, and not only with the cure of disease. The doctor must attend to health maintenance and not only to treatment or even prevention of specific diseases. He should no longer look befuddled when a patient asks him, "Doctor, what regimen do you suggest in order that I may remain healthy?" This implies, of course, changes in medical orientation that in turn imply changes in medical education both difficult to design in detail and not easy to institute in practice. But again we have not seriously thought about how to do this because we have not seen that it was something that might need doing. To recognize and identify this problem is to take the first, and thus the biggest, step toward its amelioration.

I am not saying that doctors should cease to be concerned about disease or that they should keep us in hospitals and clinics until we become fully healthy. I do suggest that physicians should be more interested than they are in finding ways to keep us from their doors. Though medicine must remain in large part restorative and remedial, greater attention to healthy functioning and to regimens for becoming and remaining healthy could be very salutary, even toward the limited goal of reducing the incidence of disease. Little intelligence and imagination have thus far been expended by members of the profession or by health insurance companies to devise incentive schemes that would reward such a shift in emphasis (e.g., that would reward financially both patient and physician if the patient stays free of the need for the latter's services). I invite people cleverer than I to make such efforts, especially in conjunction with the likely changes in the financing of medical care.

If we turn from these aspects of doctoring to the subject of medical research, we enter an area much more directly affected by government policy. (Roughly two-thirds of the biomedical research done in the United States is supported by federal funds.) It is an old story that what is honored by the polity will be practiced there, and it is the medical research of today, reflecting the hopes and fears of our representatives, that will shape the medical practice of tomorrow. What kind of medical research should we be supporting or supporting more vigorously than at present? The foregoing arguments all point to the importance of epidemiological research on *healthiness*. We need to devise better indices of healthiness than mortality and morbidity statistics which, I have argued, are in fact not indices of *health* at all. The studies like those of Breslow and his collaborators are a step in the right direction and should be encouraged. Only with better measures of healthiness can we really evaluate the results of our various health practices and policies.

We also need large-scale epidemiological research into health maintenance to learn more about what promotes health and what undermines it. More sophisticated studies in nutrition, bodily exercise, rest and sleep, relaxation, and responses to stress could be very useful, as could expanded research into personal habits of health and hygiene and their effects on general healthiness, overall resistance to disease, and specific resistance to specific diseases. We need to identify and learn about such healthy subgroups in the community as the Mormons and to discover what accounts for their success. All of these things are probably obvious, and most of them have been championed for years by people in public health and preventive medicine—though they too have placed the greater weight on disease prevention than on health maintenance. Their long-ignored advice is finally beginning to be heeded with promising results. For example, a recent study reports a surprising downturn (after a twenty-five year climb) in the death rate from heart attacks among middle-aged men, attributed in part to changes in smoking and eating habits and to new treatments for high blood pressure. Yet this approach will always seem banal and pedestrian in comparison with the glamorous and dramatic style of high-technology therapeutics with the doctor locked in mortal combat with overt disease, displaying his marvelous and magical powers. My high regard for these powers cannot stifle the question whether the men who first suggested adding chlorine to drinking water or invented indoor plumbing didn't contribute more to healthiness than the Nobel Prize winners in medicine and physiology who discovered the chemical wonders of enzyme structure or of vision. It might be worthwhile to consider by what kinds of incentives and rewards the National Institutes of Health or the AMA might encourage more and better research into health maintenance and disease prevention.

Yet as has been repeatedly emphasized, doctors and public health officials have only limited power to improve our health. Health is not a commodity which can be delivered. Medicine can help only those who help themselves. Discovering what will promote and maintain health is only half the battle; we must find ways to promote and inculcate good health habits and to increase personal responsibility for health. This is, no doubt, the most fundamental and also the most difficult task. It is but one more instance of that age-old challenge: how to get people to do what is good for them without tyrannizing them. The principles of freedom and of wisdom do not always—shall I say, do not very often?—lead in the same direction. Since this is not a new difficulty, we do have some experience in how to think about it. Consider the problem of getting people to obey the law. Policemen and judges are clearly needed to handle the major crimes and criminals, but it would be foolish to propose—and dangerous to provide—even that degree of police surveillance and interference required to prevent only the most serious lawbreaking. But though justice is the business of the policeman and the judge, it is not their business alone. Education—at home, in schools, in civic and religious institutions—can "teach" law-abidingness far better than policemen can, and where the former is successful there is less need of the latter.

Yet even without considering the limitations of this analogy, the limits of the power of teachers—and of policemen as well—to produce law-abidingness are all too apparent. And when one considers that fear of immediate, identifiable punishment probably deters lawbreaking more than fear of unhealth deters sloth and gluttony, we see that we face no simple task. The wages of poor health habits during youth are paid only much later, so much later that it is difficult to establish the relation of cause and effect, let alone to make it vivid enough to influence people's actions. If it isn't likely to rain for twenty years, few of us are likely to repair and maintain our leaky roofs.

This is not a counsel of despair. On the contrary, I am much impressed with the growing interest in health and health education in recent years, including the greater concern for proper nutrition, adequate exercise, dental hygiene, and the hazards of smoking, and with the evidence that at least among some groups this attention is bearing fruit. Nevertheless, when we consider the numerous impediments to setting in order our lives and our communities, I think we should retain a healthy doubt about just how healthy we Americans are likely, as a community, to become.

This skepticism is rather lacking in most political pronouncements and policies regarding health. Making unwarranted inferences from medicine's past successes against *infectious* disease, being excessively impressed with the technological brilliance of big-hospital medicine, mobilizing crusades and crash programs against cancer and heart disease, the health politicians speak as if more money, more targeted research, better distribution of services, more doctors and hospitals, and bigger and better cobalt machines, lasers, and artificial organs will bring the medical millennium to every American citizen. Going along with all this is a lack of attention to health maintenance and patient responsibility. While it would surely be difficult for the federal government to teach responsibility, we should not be pleased when its actions in fact discourage responsibility.

One step in this direction is the growing endorsement of the so-called right to health beyond the already ambiguous and dubious right to health care. A recent article argues thus:

The right to *health* is a fundamental right. It expresses the profound truth that a person's autonomy and freedom rest upon his ability to function physically and psychologically. It asserts that no other person can, with moral justification, deprive him of that ability. The right to *health care* or the right to *medical care*, on the other hand, are qualified rights. They flow from the fundamental right, but are implemented in institutions and practices only when such are possible and reasonable and only when other rights are not thereby impeded. (Italics in original. Lee and Jonsen 1974, pp. 591–92.)[3]

If the right to health means only the right not to have one's health destroyed by another, then it is a reasonable but rather impotent claim in the health care arena; the right to health care or medical care could hardly flow from a right to health unless the right to health meant also and mainly the right to become and to be kept healthy. But if health is what we say it is, it is an unlikely subject of a right in either sense. Health is a state of being, not something that can be given, and only in indirect ways is it something that can be taken away or undermined by other human beings. It no more makes sense to claim a right to health than to claim a right to wisdom or courage. These excellences of body and of soul require natural gift, attention, effort, and discipline on the part of each person who desires them. To make my health someone else's duty is not only unfair; it is to impose a duty impossible to fulfill. Though I am not particularly attracted by the language of rights and duties in regard to health, I would lean much more in the direction, once traditional, of saying that health is a *duty*, that one has an obligation to preserve one's own health. The theory of a right to health flies in the face of good sense, serves to undermine personal responsibility, and in addition places obligation where it cannot help but be unfulfillable.

Similarly, the amendment to the Medicare legislation which provides payment for "kidney-machine" treatment for all in need at a cost from $10,000 to $40,000 per patient is, for all its good intentions, a questionable step. First of all, it establishes the principle that the federal government is the savior of last resort—or, as is more likely at this price tag, the savior of first resort—for specific persons with specific diseases. In effect, the government has said that it is in the national interest for the government to pay, disease by disease, life by life, for lifesaving measures for all its citizens. The justice of providing benefits of this magnitude solely to people with kidney disease has been loudly questioned and hemophilia organizations are pressing for government financing of comparably expensive treatment. Others have called attention to the impossible financial burden that the just extension of this coverage would entail. Finally, this measure gives governmental endorsement in a most dramatic and visible way to the high-cost, technological, therapy-oriented approach to health. This approach has been challenged, on the basis of a searching analysis of this kidney-machine legislation, in a report by a panel of the Institute of Medicine (1973) of the National Academy of Sciences which, with admirable self-restraint, comments: "One wonders how many billions of dollars the nation would now be spending on iron lungs if research for the cure of polio had not been done."

This is not to say that, in the particular case of the kidney machines and under the special circumstances in which the legislation was passed, a persuasive case was not made on the other side. Clearly it was hoped that perfection of kidney transplantation or future prevention of kidney disease would make this high-cost insurance obsolete before too long. Moreover, no one wishes to appear to be—or, indeed, to be—callous about the loss of life, especially preventable and premature loss of life. Still the dangers of the kidney-machine legislation must be acknowledged.

One might even go so far as to suggest that prudent and wise legislators and policymakers must in the future resist (in a way that no private doctor should be permitted to resist) the temptation to let compassion for individual calamities and general sentimentality rule in these matters. Pursuing the best health policy for the American people—that is, a policy to encourage and support their best possible health—may indeed mean *not* taking certain measures that would prevent known deaths. Only by focusing on health and how one gets it, and by taking a more long-range view, can our health policy measure up in deed to its good intentions.

The proposals for national health insurance seem also to raise difficulties of this sort and more. Medical care is certainly very expensive and therefore, for this reason alone, not equally available to all. The economic problems are profound and genuine and there are few dispassionate observers who are not convinced that something needs to be done. Many technical questions have been debated and discussed, including the range of coverage and the sources of financing, and organized medicine has voiced its usual concern regarding governmental interference, a concern which I have already indicated I share in regard to the delimitation of the doctor's role and the scope of health care. But some of the most serious issues have received all too little attention.

Proposals for national health insurance take for granted the wisdom of our current approaches to the pursuit of health and thereby insure that in the future we will get more of the same. The proposals will simply make available to the noninsured what the privately insured now get: a hospital-centered, highly technological, disease-oriented, therapy-centered medical care. The proposals have entirely ignored the question of whether what we now do in health is what we *should* be doing. They not only endorse the status quo, but fail to take advantage of the rare opportunity which financial crises provide to reexamine basic questions and directions. The irony is that real economizing in health care is probably possible only by radically reorienting the pursuit of health.

One cannot help getting the impression that it is economic *equality*, not health and not even economizing, that is the primary aim of these proposals. Indeed, many of these proposals ought rather to be called "National Financial Disaster Insurance," for their relation to health is rather incidental. At a recent seminar in which I participated, an official of HEW informally expressed irritation at those who are questioning whether the so-called health care delivery system is really making us healthier and suggested that their main goal was to undermine liberal programs enacted in recent years. Yet this official went on to say that even if the evidence conclusively showed that all the government's health programs in no way actually improved health, the programs ought to be continued for their extra-medical—i.e., social and economic—benefits. For myself, I confess that I would prefer as my public health official the cold-hearted, even mean-spirited fellow who is interested in health and who knows how to promote it.

All the proposals for national health insurance embrace without qualification the no-fault principle. They therefore choose to ignore the importance of personal responsibility for the state of one's health or to treat it as irrelevant. As a result, they pass up an opportunity to build both positive and negative inducements into the insurance payment plan by, for example, refusing or reducing benefits for chronic respiratory disease care to persons who continue to smoke or by reducing coinsurance premiums for people who enroll in physical fitness programs or who keep their weight down.

There are, of course, complicated questions of justice raised here, and even to suggest that the sick ever be in any way blamed or penalized flies in the face of current custom and ways of thinking. Yet one need not be a Calvinist or a Spartan to see merit in the words of a wise physician, Robert S. Morison, writing on much the same subject:

In the perspectives of today, cardiovascular illness in middle age not only runs the risk of depriving families of their support, or society of certain kinds of services; it increasingly places on society the obligation to spend thousands of dollars on medical care to rescue an individual from the results of a faulty living pattern. Under these conditions, one wonders how much longer we can go on talking about a right to health without some balancing talk about the individual's responsibility to keep healthy.

I am told that Thorstein Veblen used to deplore the fact that in California they taxed the poor to send the rich to college. One wonders how he would react to a system which taxes the virtuous to send the improvident to hospital. (Morison 1974, p. 4.)

But even leaving aside questions of justice and looking only at the pursuit of health, one has reason to fear that the new insurance plan, whichever one it turns out to be, may actually contribute to a worsening rather than an improvement in our nation's health, especially if there is no balancing program to encourage individual responsibility for health maintenance.

One final word. Despite all that I have said, I would emphasize that health, while a good, cannot be the greatest good either for an individual or for a community. Politically, an excessive preoccupation with health can conflict with the pursuit of other social and economic goals (e.g., when cancer-phobia leads to governmental regulations that unreasonably restrict industrial activity or personal freedom). But more fundamentally, it is not mere life, nor even a healthy life, but rather a good and worthy life for which we must aim. And while poor health may weaken our efforts, good health alone is an insufficient condition or sign of a worthy human life. Indeed, though there is no such thing as being too healthy, there *is* such a thing as being too concerned about health. To be preoccupied with the body is to neglect the soul, for which we should indeed care "first and most" and more than we now do. We must strike a proper balance, a balance that can only be furthered if the approach to health also concentrates on our habits of life.

2

THOMAS C. SCHELLING

Government and Health*

The health industry—its production, consumption, and regulation. The financial aspects of government health programs. Characteristics of health care insurance. Incentives to lower insurance costs. The problem of insuring the poor.

How do we *want* to define the government's role and responsibility in the health of its citizens? They are for us to define to meet our wants—not something to be discovered through philosophical inquiry or by searching our constitutional traditions for some basic "right" that is ready to be discovered.

*Adapted from the author's paper prepared for the Institute of Medicine's Annual Meeting November 5–6, 1975; reprinted with the permission of the Institute of Medicine (National Academy of Science, Institute of Medicine, Washington, DC).

Medical care alone in this country—and medical care does not include all activities related to health—is more than $100 billion per year of producing and spending, or $500 per capita, and getting larger. Whatever the government does, it will be spending *our* money and regulating the hospitals and clinics that *we* pay for and influencing *our* consumption of eggs, alcohol, and tobacco; helping us at each other's expense in extremity, infirmity, and old age; and doing it with money that might otherwise be spent on schools, prisons, and cleaner water or that we might instead spend individually on food, housing, or horse races.

Most of us, not just at a meeting of the Institute of Medicine but in this country, are going to pay for what we get from the government. The government is not some independent source of benefits; it's our representatives deciding how to spend our money. And a lot of our money is at stake.

Some of us are too poor to pay our share, some are too clever to pay our taxes, some are too sick to do anything but ask for help, and some may be too healthy to care very much. But most of us should be thinking about how best to use the facilities and processes of government in order to do in the area of health and medicine what we don't manage to do very well or very equitably by ourselves.

THREE AREAS OF RESPONSIBILITY

I find it useful to divide this large area of potential responsibility into three quite distinct parts. One is the *production* side of the health industry: doctors and nurses, hospitals and clinics, drugs and dentures and eyeglasses, nursing homes and ambulances. This is $100 billion per year of human and material resources. It is $100 billion per year of incomes earned in the provision of health care. It is the schooling, the licensing, the regulating, the ethics and self-regulation, the cheating and tax evasion, the rescuing and comforting and lifesaving. This is the few million people who serve—in hospitals and factories and clinics and laundries and doctors' offices and drugstores—the two hundred million or so who sooner or later need care or medicine. The second area of governmental concern can be characterized in either of two ways. We can call it the *consuming* public, meaning all those two hundred million people who from time to time, in unequal and often unexpected amounts, receive the $100 billion per year of care and treatment and medicine. We usually think of them as the sick and the injured, the pregnant, the dying, the hypochondriacs, the allergic, the congenitally defective who need eyeglasses and other more serious help, and the people who are careless about their teeth or diet. Or we can characterize this side of the market as the people who *pay* for that $100 billion worth of medical care—paying out of our earnings or assets or going into debt; paying directly or through taxes or insurance premiums or charitable contributions, and sometimes through the prices of things whose production costs include medical fringe benefits.

For many purposes it is important to distinguish the consumers from the payers. But it is good to remind ourselves that we are the same population. Only some of us are sick now; but most of us get sick eventually and we are all at risk. Only some of us are elderly but most of us hope to be. If we think not of individuals at a moment but of families and lifetimes, most of us consume a good deal of medical care and most of us pay for medical care, our own or somebody else's.

Furthermore, these two ways of characterizing the consuming and paying public correspond to two concerns that most of us have about medical care. One concern is with the *quality* and *availability* of the care. The other is with its *expense*. People complain of poor treatment or lack of treatment and people complain of the high cost of becoming sick or injured or incapacitated. The complaints about quality and availability emanate from the consuming public but are directed at the producing side of the medical-care market. The government's role and responsibility in the quality and availability of medical care are best discussed in relation to the medical-care industry. But the problem of expense is mainly a problem for the consuming public.

The *third area* of potential government role and responsibility I define in a somewhat open-ended way. It is all that the government might do about our health that is not directly related to medical care, medicine, or the treatment of people whose health is poor. I have in mind everything the government might do or might not do about the way we eat and drink and sleep and exercise and smoke: the conditions in which we work and the conditions in which we play; the air we breathe and the water we drink and the bugs that bite us and the bicycles that run into us and the noise in our ears and the drugs we abuse. The government, as represented in the school system, once made most of us exercise—often in ways we didn't like at ages when we didn't need the exercise—and gave us a little advice on how to avoid tooth decay and venereal disease. It hasn't done much for us since except to take cigarette ads off television and make our seatbelts whine when we don't put them on. There was a glorious moment in the early 1960s when the president's family publicized long walks and touch football. We lost a war against alcohol fifty years ago and a war against marijuana more recently. Altogether we have a striking lack of consensus on what the government's role should be, even on whether the government should have a role in relation to what we do that affects our own health.

A lot of what medicine can do for us it is already doing. What motivates most discussion of national health policy is how to take care of the financial consequences. But the big changes in our health seem likely to occur, if they ever do occur, from changes in the way we behave rather than changes in the way the doctors and hospitals take care of us. I haven't much to say about the government's responsibility in this but I shall return to it at the end of my chapter if only to emphasize that it deserves our attention, whether or not our attention can yet be productive.

HEALTH POLICY AS FINANCIAL POLICY

Most of what I shall say concerns the second area: the consuming and expense-paying side of the medical-care market. Most proposed governmental initiatives relate to paying for medical care. Even most of the organizational proposals are closely related to financial incentives. If we include, besides the question of who pays, the questions of how payment is made, what gets paid for, and how the costs are shared, we are at the heart of most current proposals about some kind of national health program.

What needs to be stressed, and what ought to be our point of departure for a major national medical care program, is that the problem is basically financial, not medical. The problem is money, not beds and drugs and doctors and nurses. It is that beds and doctors and hospitals and nurses and drugs are a large expense, measured against our incomes.

I have to emphasize that the financial side of national health care is not the whole field of national policy toward health and medicine. I will not even claim that it is the most important side of the problem. It is, however, a large part of the problem and the part that is best examined and planned for in its entirety rather than piecemeal. Just as the federal government has a multiplicity of programs relating to employment and manpower but a substantially integrated system of unemployment compensation, so the government may need a variety of decentralized programs to cope with the producing side of the health-care economy but an integrated approach to the financial side. The two sides interact importantly, because the financial arrangements can provide leverage on the production side and because bad financial incentives can seriously interfere with the efficient organization of the producing side. But no integrated financial program can hope to cover all the activities and responsibilities of the federal government with respect to the medical-care industry and its organization nor will all governmental programs occur at the federal level.

For most of us medicine and the medical industry are complex and mysterious, even though we are continually in touch with it. How to manage medical schools and the medical and nursing professions, hospitals and the drug industry, is a set of very specialized questions, technically and economically. But once we recognize that the big urgent problem is a financial problem we are back on familiar ground. Indeed, we can almost forget that what we are dealing with is heart attacks and brain concussions and arthritis rather than poor crops and lost jobs and burned houses, and just deal with poverty, financial emergency, and financial management.

To overstate it only slightly, most proposed integrated national health programs—especially those referred to as national health insurance—are programs to cope with financial problems, not programs to cope with medical problems. The fundamental problem to which most governmental initiatives are addressed is not how to get an appendectomy for a person who has appendicitis in the middle of the night. It is how to keep the appendectomy from being a financial calamity or an unfair financial burden. If the heating system breaks down on your chicken farm you have no choice but to get it fixed or your chickens will die; if your appendix flares up you are in much the same situation. It is not that one is a heating problem and one a medical problem. Both are financial problems. You call different telephone numbers for help, but both emergencies show up on the same bank statement.

THREE ASPECTS OF THE FINANCIAL PROBLEM

It is useful to distinguish three aspects of the overall problem of medical expense. One is the medical expenses of the poor. In terms of governmental responsibility this is a big part of the problem. But in the overall organization of the financial side of the medical industry it is a significant part but not the major part.

The second and larger part is the question, what is a sensible insurance system to take care of the fact that we are all at risk but some of us have medical needs and expenses way out of proportion?

The third aspect is what kind of financial arrangements will best help to keep medical costs from rising too rapidly?

Let me postpone momentarily the problems of the poor. Those may be the problems that most concern you, but I'm going to argue that they are not the problems to which the overall structure of a national medical insurance program should be addressed. Most of a national medical insurance program will be concerned with how the majority among us, who are not poor enough to avoid substantially paying our own way, want to share the costs of our medical care.

CHARACTERISTICS OF MEDICAL INSURANCE

What is it that makes medical insurance different from other kinds of insurance—collision damage on the automobile, fire, life, hailstorm, or burglary?

Medical insurance does have features that make it appreciably different from some other kinds of insurance. A simple but important difference is that replacement cost conveniently sets an upper limit to your claim if you lost your car, your barn, your boat, or your violin. There may be disputes about what the stolen violin was worth, but the disputes will tend to be in the range of 20 to 50 percent. But if your sick body is recalcitrant and the treatment costs begin to seem endless, there is no way for the insurance company to buy you a new body at retail and dispose of the old one for salvage. If you are insured against the costs of being restored to decent health, there is no easily identified upper limit to what those costs can be.

The problem does not arise with what is sometimes called "indemnity" insurance. There are policies that pay you an amount in dollars for a broken collarbone. What you do with the money and what you do with the collarbone are not the insurer's business. Get a cheap doctor and save the difference; go to an expensive hospital and pay the excess yourself. The company gives you $400 when it sees the broken bone. Auto insurers have discovered that people settle for smaller amounts in cash than in repair services because they always want the smashed left door to look as good as new if somebody else pays for it but are often happy to get it banged back into workable shape for $50 if they can pocket $100 in cash.

Another problem with medical insurance is that society finds it difficult to deny care to people whose lives depend on care and who cannot pay for it. The Coast Guard feels obliged to help a vessel in distress; city fire departments cannot decline the calls of people whose houses are burning but who are delinquent in their property taxes. If your car is smashed or your TV stolen there is no place to go with an irresistible claim for restoration at public expense, but doctors and hospitals are not very good at evicting you from their care once you go broke. Furthermore, if medical expenses make you unable to work or too poor to support your family, public assistance may not pay your medical bills directly but may substantially redress your financial plight so that there is public expense, even though the insurance isn't called medical.

Another feature that makes medical insurance somewhat different is that the insured person is not only pretty incompetent but officially incompetent to prescribe his or her own treatment or to know what is needed. We are pretty helpless when the repairman says we need a new picture tube or universal joint, but most of us have even less choice when the doctor wants us hospitalized or prescribes some laboratory tests or drugs. By ethics and training doctors know more about medicine than they do about family budgeting, and it is hard for the doctor and his patient to reach a decision together about how much money it's worth to alleviate some pain or improve some mobility or reduce anxiety or avoid some risk of leaving orphans. It appears to be also more difficult for an insurance company to drag its feet on a doctor's prescription than to haggle over the quality of the paint job on a repaired automobile. An important characteristic of many kinds of insurance is that hazards are not uniform among the population; premiums ought therefore to differ among individuals, but insurers are poor at identifying degrees of risk and adjusting premiums accordingly. The insured individuals often know more about their own susceptibilities than an insurance company can find out. Premiums therefore tend to reflect the average level of risk; and the people who know that their own risks are greater are attracted to the good bargain that insurance represents, while the people who believe themselves to face appreciably lower risks than the average find the insurance no such good bargain unless they can document the good state of their health (or their fire protection, or their driving ability, or whatever may be involved) and qualify for lower premiums. With respect to collision damage people may go ahead and insure anyway; my impression is that people "overinsure" their automobiles. It does not appear that there is a widespread compulsive tendency to overinsure against medical expenses, and the people who consider themselves comparatively healthy—or at least those who have no serious apprehensions about illness or injury—will be less likely to participate voluntarily. (A good example is pregnancy; those who intend not to have children will be less attracted to pregnancy benefits than those who have already planned on an early birth.)

This tendency can be serious for the prospects of an insurance system. Among any potentially insured population there will be some who are less at risk than the average and know it and who may find the insurance uneconomical. In staying out they withdraw themselves from the population whose average expense they would have held down, so their nonparticipation raises the average. Now somebody else is below the higher average; if he declines to participate the average goes still higher. In order to be viable almost any insurance plan requires the participation of some people who pay higher premiums than they ought to and who may know it. After every attempt has been made to identify them objectively and to offer them selectively lower premiums, it may in the end be necessary to oblige the participation of some who would not find the insurance a worthwhile bargain in order to keep the entire enterprise from unraveling.

(The injustice in making people who consider themselves below average in risk pay a premium close to the average is not as great as it at first appears. Many who would decline insurance on grounds of good health preserve the option to change their minds. Unless they acquire some undisguisable and easily diagnosed disability, they can get into an insurance plan when their health or their environment changes in a way that makes the insurance a good bargain. They are thus getting free insurance against "uninsurability"—a benefit they were not paying for.)

There is one more characteristic of medical-care insurance that is pertinent to whether or not the government should assume responsibility for deciding whether or not people must participate. That is that some people are born into situations of poorer health than other people. The differences are partly genetic, partly family income or culture, partly location, partly plain luck. People might wish to be insured against being born into poor health. A rationally devised health-care insurance system would charge people higher premiums if they sign up with poor health prospects. The ideal time to join might be before one is conceived, so that potential infants are insured against being born into poor health and therefore being born into a high-premium bracket. There is no way to do that. But we might adopt a "social contract" in which all who are born into citizenship are covered in advance, before it is known even whose children they will be. Thus we are born with an obligation to pay the premiums, but also born eligible for insurance at the standard premium irrespective of the health prospects with which we are born.

That would make health-care insurance rather like unemployment insurance (and like the "income insurance" represented in federal welfare programs). People generally cannot avoid employment taxes by being merely so eminently employable that they have no acknowledged need for unemployment insurance. Under this philosophy the lucky people are the ones who are born healthy enough to get what in retrospect looks like a bad bargain and the unlucky ones—as with any insurance program—are those who get the most benefits.

(People could of course pay health-care insurance for their unborn children, but it would then have to be either a lifetime contract or else high-priced insurance against being declared a high-premium person at some stipulated age. This is not necessarily a responsibility so attractive that parents should appreciate being left with the decision.)

NATIONAL HEALTH INSURANCE

I reach the conclusion that at least some minimum level of universal mandatory medical-care insurance makes sense. By "minimal" I do not mean small in insured values: it's the potential catastrophes that constitute the "basic minimum."

Still leaving aside the problem of the poor, we should ask ourselves what kind of coverage and what system of premiums and what deductibles and percentage shares of "coinsurance" look like a good arrangement, remembering that whatever we get from the system we are going to pay for it. Here we are mainly dealing with incentives. Of course if I'm sick and insured and I have a chance to get better care or more privacy or air-conditioning or less pain or even better healing of a wound, I'll take all I can get if the insurance company pays for it. And so will you. And then I realize that while my cost is distributed among a million other people, a million other people are ready to share their costs with me.

COPING WITH INCENTIVES

There are several common ways of coping with incentives in the insurance business. One is to make the insured pay a fraction of all the costs he incurs, the fraction being small enough to avoid financial calamity and large enough to make him or his physician think twice before incurring any expensive treatment that is at all optional. This is called *coinsurance*. Percentages from 10 to 30 are talked about in relation to medical insurance. The coinsurance percentage needn't be uniform over all ailments and all kinds of treatments. They needn't be uniform among income levels. They needn't be uniform over the entire potential range of expenditures; 30 percent on a week's stay and 5 or 10 percent on a year's confinement might be equally effective compromises.

And *compromises* are what these are. In principle one wants to insure against the whole expense. In principle one wants strong motivation to hold expenses down. These two principles conflict. All one can look for is a pragmatic compromise.

A second feature is *deductibles*, familiar to us in automobile and household insurance as well as in medical insurance. Deductibles serve two purposes. One is to provide the full-cost incentive to economize on expenses within a range that is financially manageable. The other is to avoid the administrative costs of processing small claims. Administrative costs are worth holding down in policies that cover households and automobiles, but probably will not be so in medical care. Unlike burglaries and collisions, medical expenses tend to accumulate over time or within the family, and a lot of the record-keeping has to be done whether or not the small expenses are reimbursable. Fires, burglaries, and auto collisions are discrete events; but a protracted illness can begin with a sore throat or a backache, and it is hard to tell whether a small expense is a prelude to a larger total. Furthermore, people may not be able to control the date on which they fall down or get an infection but there is some leeway in visiting the doctor before or after New Year's Day in order to exhaust an annual deductible.

Therefore the best way to handle deductibles is not in an annual accounting period but in a manner that is more cumulative over time. Further, a deductible can be thought of as "100 percent coinsurance," and rather than have it jump suddenly from 100 percent down to 10 or 25 percent once the total reaches a particular figure, a "graduated coinsurance" system with averaging over several years would be a sensible arrangement.

A third feature that makes sense is a wider use of *indemnity insurance* . To the extent that we can approximate the customary costs of well-defined ailments and treatments, broken bones or tonsillectomies or appendectomies, at least in the absence of complications it makes sense to price them with a dollar amount. At first glance this may sound like poor medical practice, but what we're dealing with is financial practice. If your radiators burst or your favorite apple tree blows down in a hurricane or it rains on your vacation, you may have a financial claim that reduces the severity of the loss; you can do the same with a broken bone. The fact that the settlement may be too much or too little by 30 or 40 percent is too bad, especially if the settlement is too little, but to receive $300 too little for a broken bone is no worse than receiving $300 too little for a broken glass in one's store. The bone and the glass don't care and the dollars all come out of the same place.

A fourth common technique is to provide incentives for the avoidance of damage by *lowering premiums* for policyholders who take precautions that will reduce risks. (A currently popular example is the auto bumper that reduces collision damage.) There have been imaginative proposals to give "merit-rated" premium reductions to people who do not smoke, who avoid overweight, or who can document some kind of regular exercise; less imaginative but more practical may be modest premium reductions for people who get periodic examinations, but whether there is more to be accomplished here than merely to dramatize personal health care has not been established as far as I know. It is an area that invites research but does not yet offer promise.

A fifth way to hold costs down is to avoid those perverse *criteria for reimbursement* that actually invite exaggerated expense. If hospitalization determines eligibility for treatments like oral surgery that could be accomplished in an office or clinic, physicians cannot help saving their patients' money by occasionally prescribing unnecessarily expensive treatment. It has to be acknowledged that there may be a good reason for reimbursing, say, certain kinds of therapy that are institutionalized in a hospital setting, but those reasons have to be scrutinized to make sure the effect is not merely to elevate the level and cost of treatment. Nursing homes and home-care centers appear to be important examples.

A sixth feature of some insurance—one receiving increasing attention in the field of medical care—is incentives on the *provider* of the care. (A homely analogy is the laundry that offers white-shirt subscriptions: the subscriber checks out shirts his own size and returns them to the laundry, never owning his own shirts. The laundry is motivated to handle the shirts with care because the savings accrue to the laundry.) There are experiments with prepaid medical systems and "health maintenance organizations" that are simultaneously responsible for providing the care and paying for it, their own reimbursement being from regular payments unrelated to the actual provision of care. The principle is a sound one. It is also good reason for allowing diversity and experimentation in the way medical insurance is organized, and for not getting locked into a rigidly uniform system of insurance.

A final point, not so much a feature of the insurance as a matter of coverage, is that as much as possible should be *excluded* from insurance on grounds that a lot of expenses average out within the family or over a lifetime or are not big enough to be worth the administrative cost and waste of insurance. Eyeglasses are an example. There is no more reason to be insured for eyeglasses than to be insured for shoes. Children can't go to school without eyeglasses, but they can't go to school without shoes either. Shoes and eyeglasses cost the same kind of money. In general, the expenses that tend to be regular, predictable, and not bunched in time have no business in an insurance scheme. Ruthless exclusion of things to which the insurance principle doesn't apply is one of the best ways of putting the full incentive back on the customer to shop around and economize with remarkably little addition to total hardship.

INSURANCE FOR THE POOR

Now the poor. By the poor I mean the people who are not expected to pay their way in an insurance scheme and, in gatherings like those of the Institute of Medicine, the people toward whom we feel an obligation to provide at our own expense some of the things they need that they can't pay for. Descriptively we might want to make some reference to the elderly here, since the elderly are often poor and usually have no future earnings to borrow against. The elderly have especially large medical needs. While "poor" describes their financial status, "elderly" is part of the image to keep in mind.

The important thing about the poor in health insurance is that the problem is mainly money, not medicine. That is, the reason we distinguish the poor from the rich is primarily that they get the same ailments and need the same treatments and incur the same expenses, and have much less money to pay for them. There are other categories of the population for which the problem is not purely financial. Children, convicts, lighthouse keepers, some of the mentally ill, and people who don't speak English may all have problems that are not basically financial. But here we are discussing the financial problems of the poor in relation to their medical needs.

Notice: the problem is *not* that they can't afford protracted treatment or intensive care or technologies. It is not that a heart attack and hospitalization is a greater burden on a poor person than on somebody who is well-to-do. The problem is not that some of us can afford brain surgery and some of us are too poor. No, that's the problem we solve with a national medical insurance plan. Under a national medical insurance plan, the problem of the poor is that they have *an annual premium to pay that they think or we think is too large* .

And we have a rough idea of what those costs are. Private-patient care per capita is currently around $450 per year. Part of that annual cost should be outside any insurance scheme. Part of it represents the better care and comfort that some people can afford and others can't. There is no reason to think that the poor want to live like the rich when they go to the hospital and then go home to a slum or ghetto if they have any choice in the kinds of benefits that they get at public expense. So we are probably talking about $200 per capita as the extra average annual cost that the poor might incur if they paid their own way in an insurance program that gave them most but not all of what the well-to-do enjoy when they get sick.

Two hundred dollars apiece per year is a lot of money for a poor family. But it is also a lot of rent money for a poor family, food money, day-care help for the children while the mother works.

This is where the question arises: should the poor—those who do not pay their own way in a medical insurance plan—receive less care and comfort and medical attention than those who are not poor and who pay their own way? My answer is yes, they should receive less, because they cannot afford equal care *even at public expense* . They cannot afford it because there are other things they need at public expense besides medical care and there are limits to what they can get at public expense. Cities and states right now are facing hard choices among medicines and medical care, direct welfare benefits, nursing-home laundry services, and police protection for the poor. To provide the poor, as a matter of principal, the same level of medical service as the rest of the population wants to provide for itself is an evasion of the fact that they are poor and have urgent unattended other needs too.

It probably doesn't matter terribly just how we charge people for their medical insurance at different levels of income, the very poor and the not-so-poor and the well-to-do. It doesn't matter much for the reason I have been stressing all along. Money is money. We can subsidize their medical insurance, or give them food stamps and let them pay their medical insurance, or reduce their taxes. If they have to belong and do belong to a national medical insurance program, we are out of the medical business and back in the poverty business. The question is not what to do about medical insurance for the poor. It is what to do about their being poor.

If we had a completely nationalized medical insurance scheme, which I think we do not want, it really wouldn't make any difference whether we charged everybody an insurance premium related to his income, or allowed for it all in the income tax and welfare benefits. If I were to pay for every member of my family in a federal medical insurance program, I wouldn't much care whether I wrote a larger check to the Internal Revenue Service or a separate check to the Social Security Administration.

I think that the financing of medical insurance is important because we do not want a completely nationalized scheme. We want to allow room for experimentation—perhaps different arrangements in different states, different arrangements for people who like health maintenance organizations, and so forth. But the problem of the poor is a problem of taxes and welfare and poverty. It is not a problem that has to be thought of in the medical context, once we have decided that everybody has to have some kind of insurance against major medical expenses.

So much for the subject of a national health insurance program. I think that subject is reaching its climax. We are likely to have some kind of national program within a few years. And although the program will be forever controversial and subject to change and experiment, and it won't solve the problem of medical organization, at least it will settle the major issues that have dominated the field of federal health policy for the past decade or more.

3

ARTHUR SELDON

The Lessons of Centralized Medicine

Centralized health care in some other nations. Great Britain's National Health Service—a Mad Hatter's teaparty. The political dilemma of centralized medicine. The gulf between government and private services—price problems and the 1975–1976 crisis. Government cost-sharing in Canada. The need for patients to share health insurance. "Politician, heal thyself."

FROM CENTRAL FINANCING
TO CENTRAL CONTROL

National health insurance (NHI) centralizes the financing of medical care through taxation and/or social insurance. (The difference between them is insignificant if payment to doctors and hospitals is made by government agency rather than by patients.) As a financing mechanism NHI does not centralize control of health care by nationalizing hospitals, clinics, etc., and directly employing personnel. Under NHI health care—at least the very large part of it comprising personal services rather than public goods—could continue to be supplied in private hospitals and by family doctors (and others) paid by capitation or by fee.* It could; the question is whether under NHI it would.

Health services around the world are supplied by varying combinations of government and private financing and control. Where can the United States look for the most relevant experience and lessons?

The only country of comparable size and population is the Soviet Union where—except for occasional official forms of "private" medicine (pay polyclinics in some towns for second opinions) and more common unofficial black markets in which patients pay for better care than the state can supply—the government both finances and controls health services. Government can promote health by encouraging or requiring regular exercise, directing doctors to remote areas, and other devices. But if the purpose is to improve health services while retaining some measure of free choice by patients and doctors, paternalistic or authoritarian medical systems do not have much to teach in general principle, although there may be technical details to emulate. The overriding aim is the best health that can be obtained from given resources, not the best health no matter what the cost in education, housing, defense, or freedom.

In the smaller, less brittle, more "liberal" communist societies such as Czechoslovakia, Hungary, Yugoslavia, and Poland, where economists in touch with the West have more influence, fees are occasionally levied to discourage overprescribing and informal payment between patient and doctor is variously tolerated.

---

*Capitation involves an annual payment per patient, while fee limits payment to services actually rendered.

The Western but only partially industrialized countries—Italy, Spain, and Portugal—are not comparable, and the countries of South America, Africa, and Asia are even less so. None have any important lessons for national health insurance in the United States.

Then there is a group of countries more like the United States in social and economic development but with apparently better health records: Sweden, Norway, Denmark, Switzerland, and others. They are either much smaller than the United States, culturally and racially more homogeneous, or have lower living standards that restrict the personal excesses in eating, drinking, driving, etc., which cause ill health and death. Moreover, the comparison of health records by statistics of mortality and morbidity is often inconclusive; they differ in definition of "death," "stillborn," "foetal life"; records are more complete in some countries than in others; social mixes differ; the ability to act on medical advice or to accept treatment varies; and so on. World Health Organization (WHO) figures are supplied by governments and should be taken with a pinch of salt.

Several larger countries—France and Germany—are more comparable economically but have mixed systems of private government financing and control of medical care and a pricing structure for services reimbursed from insurance.

Canada has adopted elements of national insurance and is economically and culturally perhaps the most comparable country; but Canada is much smaller in population and her experience of centralized financing is short.

The United Kingdom is another country where the urge to innovate began early in the Industrial Revolution but has been diluted by social and economic theories that taught the attractions of security and communal effort. Income per head in Great Britain is now perhaps half that in the United States. But Britain has considerable experience with centralized financing and control of medical care, and for that reason the British experience contains important lessons for all Americans con-

cerned about the impact of national health insurance on the
health care delivery system in the United States.

STATE MEDICINE—PROMISE 1946, PERFORMANCE 1976

To analyze the working of NHI in practice, in contrast to the
claims and expectations, it is essential to study not only its tech-
nical/economic methods which preoccupy the protagonists but
also the political environment: the day-to-day influences and
pressures in making and executing policy. A unique insight into
both aspects is yielded by comparing the hopes for the British
National Health Service (NHS) of the Minister of Health in
1946 with the appraisal almost thirty years later of the Minister
of Health at the end of 1975. The comparison will reveal the political motives and methods in running NHS, countering criticism, and gradually tightening the government control over
medicine.

The promises were heralded by the so-called architect of
NHS, Mr. Aneurin Bevan, in opening the Second Reading
debate on the NHS bill on 30 April 1946. He asked the House of
Commons to turn from sectional interests to the "requirements
of the British people as a whole" and to eschew paper plans
based on abstract principles to "the concrete requirements of the
actual situation as it exists." (Both parts of this preamble contain dialectical flaws that confused thought in the following thirty years to the present day: below.)

The arguments for state medicine in Britain in 1946 are
echoed in the arguments for national health insurance in
America in 1979. The National Health Service, said Bevan, was
necessary because "money ought not to be permitted to stand in
the way"; no one should be "financially deterred from seeking
medical assistance at the earliest possible stage"; everyone
should "be able to receive medical and hospital help without
being involved in financial anxiety."

The pre–1946 national health insurance scheme, said Bevan, excluded the self-employed and the families of dependents because they were not insured. It did not support the family doctor with specialist services which he had to provide himself and which were often not available to the poor. Hospitals had grown up "with no plan, with no system." It was unevenly distributed: the best facilities were where they were "least needed." Many hospitals were too small to be efficient.

Moreover, British teeth were "a national reproach"; because dental treatment had to be paid for it was not demanded sufficiently, so there was a "woeful shortage" of dentists. Seventy-five percent of the people had to pay for spectacles and eye-testing. There was insufficient attention to deafness and hardly any to cheap hearing aids. Mental health was isolated from general medicine.

All these disabilities would be dealt with by the new system he proposed: a universal health service "without any insurance qualification of any sort . . . available to the whole population freely." The intention also was "to universalise the best . . . to generalise the best health advice and treatment. . . . We shall promise every citizen in this country the same standard of service." There would be "no limitation" on the assistance "given the general practitioner, the specialist, the hospitals, eye treatment, spectacles, dental treatment, hearing facilities. . . . All these are to be made available free."

"For a while" there would be some limitations. Shortage of dentists would require "us" (the government) to give priority to expectant and nursing mothers, children and later ("we hope") adolescents, but "finally" he hoped to build up a dental service for the whole population. The shortage of nurses and hospital beds meant that "it would be some time" before universal medical service could "fructify." Nevertheless this was "the object of the scheme."

It was "repugnant" for hospitals to rely on private charity, so "the voluntary hospitals must be taken over." Investigation has shown that the "proper" hospital unit should comprise about

1,000 beds, so hospitals would be "pooled, linked together," for which purpose they should "submit themselves to proper organisation." Local authorities were too small and poor for this purpose so "I decided . . . to create an entirely new hospital service" by taking over all hospitals, voluntary (independent, private) and municipal (local government). Regional hospital boards, it had been indicated by "investigations" and "advice," were the solution because they would combine hospital planning with administration.

The family doctor would (as a self-employed independent) sell his services under contract with a new body—the local executive council—half of which would comprise doctors, dentists, and chemists (retail pharmacists), under lay control to avoid syndicalism. Family doctors would be "redistributed throughout the country" to equalize densities, and sale and purchase of practices would be abolished. "I will deal with [the] opposition." Doctors would be compensated for hardship.

A doctor new to an area would apply to the local executive council for permission to practice and the Medical Practices Committee, a mainly professional body, would approve or refuse the appointment by judging "whether there were sufficient general practitioners in that area." This was not direction of doctors: "no profession should be allowed to enter the public service in a place where it is not needed." By this "negative control" Bevan hoped "over a number of years" to bring about "a positive redistribution" of family doctors.

Bevan did not favor a full salaried service: payment should reward zeal and there should be "punishment for lack of it": therefore capitation would remain the basic method of payment. But a salary would be used to help young doctors build practices, attract doctors into unattractive areas, and reward special acquirements. And fees could be charged to patients not on the NHS "panel" (lists). Here Bevan showed more understanding of human nature and market processes than his whole-hogging supporters. To outlaw fees would be "impracticable. . . . To do so would be to create a black market." There was also some regard for individual freedom and choice, at least with second opinions. "There ought to be nothing to prevent anyone having advice from another doctor . . . than his own." But this civilized insight was soon constricted by politics. It would be "unreasonable" for a patient to pay a better doctor a fee the patient could avoid simply by transferring to him. So fee payment must be small: there was danger to the state system in allowing choice of doctor and payment: "if the amount of fee paying is great, the system will break down, because the whole purpose . . . is to provide free treatment with no fee paying at all." And the same principle applied to the hospitals.

Bevan "hoped" that everyone would be on a doctor's panel, and since patients could change doctors there would not be much fee paying. But of course human nature was obstinate and might disturb the well-laid plans of political men in framing health services; "idiosyncracies are prevalent. . . . There is no reason" to stop a patient who wanted to consult another doctor. (He did not foresee the later attitude of NHS supporters who think fee paying immoral and will strike, threaten strikes, to prevent it.)

Yet Bevan saw that the market was not repressible in hospitalization. He had probably never heard of Böhm-Bawerk's teaching that economic law was stronger than government, but he had more native intelligence than his followers who wanted to suppress every health activity outside the state system: "We are driven inevitably to this fact, that unless we permit some fee paying in the public hospitals, there will be a rash of nursing homes all over the country." The NHS, said Bevan, should provide amenities or privacy or other services people wanted so that they would not wish to pay for them elsewhere; but for a time, while hospital facilities were "inadequate, . . . some people will want to buy something more than the general health service is providing." We can see clearly now, but Bevan did not then, that this interim was not short but permanent. As income rises, the gap between what people will want and what the state system can provide would not narrow but widen.

Perhaps surprisingly for an egalitarian, Bevan went even further: "Behind this there is a principle of some importance. *If the state owned a theatre it would not charge the same prices for the different seats.*" (My italics.) Let us pause. The governing party rank and file listening to Bevan reacted unhappily to its high priest acknowledging sin in the idiosyncratic citizen and taxpayer who would not resignedly accept what the state would try to supply equally for all. But the politicians lay not far below the surface in his illustration: "The state will provide a certain standard of dentistry free, but if a person wants to have his teeth filled with gold, the state will not provide that." Patients would come to want more mundane "extras" than gold.

Health centers, said the minister, would be encouraged; they would raise the general standard of the medical profession as a whole. Doctors would practice there "with great facilities." As with other NHS services, it would be "some time" before they were established everywhere. (They were established painfully slowly.) There is some affinity between health centers and health maintenance organizations (HMOs) in the United States.

The promises were repeated in a bombastic peroration:

Neither [the good doctor] nor his patient will have any financial anxiety arising out of illness. . . .

Academic medical education will be more free in the future than it has been in the past. . . .

[The NHS] will place this country in the forefront of all countries of the world in medical services. . . .

[It] will lift the shadow from millions of homes. . . .

It will keep very many people alive who might otherwise be dead. . . .

It will produce higher standards for the medical profession.

Thirty years later than Mr. Bevan, a minister of health cast in much the same philosophic/collectivist mould, Mrs. Barbara Castle, "revisited" NHS to assess its problems and achievements.

Bevan's euphoria contrasted with Castle's defensiveness: "the way things have been going in recent months it might have seemed as if there could soon be no NHS to visit at all." Consultants and junior hospital doctors had taken "industrial" action (working to rule, banning overtime, striking) as a climax to "a wave of unrest." Mrs. Castle had therefore been forced to ask herself "some pretty fundamental questions" about NHS in the face of "this wrecking mood."

This mood, she said, was "remarkable" (she meant surprising, unexpected, vexing) because NHS expenditure in 1973–1974 had reached a new "high" of 5.4 percent of the gross national product (GNP) compared with 4.0 percent in 1948. (There was no reference to other countries.) Manpower had also reached a new peak of 55,000 doctors in England and Wales against 35,000 in 1948. (There was no reference to quality.) Places in medical schools had expanded by 22 percent from 2,700 in 1970 to 3,300 in 1974 (but was the 1970 figure the optimum?). Nurses were 320,000 compared with 160,000 in 1948. (Of what standard? For how many patients? Requiring what sort of care—geriatric? psychiatric? acute? chronic?) "Despite these remarkable advances the mood of crisis—as against the reality—continues. If we are to analyse its cause we must go back into history."

Mrs. Castle's review of the bad old days before NHS will be familiar to Americans in the interpretation of recent American history presented by the advocates of national health insurance. The common people had to manage as best they could on a "patchwork" of government, municipal, and voluntary services. Many were not covered by government or private insurance. Bevan had woven "this variegated provision into a comprehensive system of health care for everyone 'from the cradle to the grave,' a system financed *and therefore regulated* by the State." (My italics.) Mrs. Castle was blurting out truths that more devious intelligences would have suppressed or rephrased.

Mrs. Castle proclaimed Bevan's "genius" for evolving "a revolutionary new formula unparalleled in the non-Communist world" (generalizing the best) which a British Medical Association (BMA) commission had advocated during the war. (Here are two further revealing aspects of state medicine: its origin in wartime Britain and Britain's unique distinction—or aberration, according to taste—as the only non-Communist Western country with state medicine.) The minister of 1946, said the minister in 1976, clearly saw the implications. First, to be comprehensive, "the Service" (a very totalitarian description) had to be financed by taxation. Second, "to universalise the best" hospitals, consultants would have to be salaried: *This would mean the nationalisation of hospitals.*" (My italics.) Third, since family doctors "dreaded a whole time salaried service" they would remain independent, self-employed, contracting with the state (through local executive councils) for capitation, with a small basic salary to help young doctors build practices.

All three "implications" are relevant to the U.S. debate on national health insurance. If the assumption is accepted that access to medical care should be divorced from personal payment, national health insurance will be found to have gaps, anomalies, and loopholes that could easily be removed by taxation with no nonsense about individual contributions and claims. And once medical care is financed by taxation it is a short step to argue that it should be organized by the state.

First, the gaps and loopholes argument can be plausible. Mrs. Castle recounted that on a visit to the United States at Easter 1975 she had found that "the dramatic increase in unemployment" had provoked "a major crisis in their health care system": workers unemployed were not covered and the federal government was having to consider emergency legislation. (Occasional unemployment *per se* is hardly an argument for state medicine; people can save, or can be helped to save, against a rainy day.)

Second, that universalization of "the best" requires nationalization will also seem persuasive if the initial aim of "free" access is accepted uncritically. Here Bevan was advised by a doctors' leader, the president of the Royal College of Physicians, that the best consultants could be induced into the lesser provincial hospitals if they were amply salaried. Bevan considered that only the state could pay enough, *and that meant state ownership of hospitals.* So he nationalized them, an act described by a doctor as "the greatest seizure of property since Henry VIII confiscated the monasteries." (Government hospitals and their flavor of orderly institutionalism will be known to Americans in war.) Third, step by step the *de jure* capitation "independent contractors" have become increasingly dependent *de facto* on state monies. The salary element has increased, with state loans and grants for premises and equipment. Mrs. Castle described Bevan's solution as insuring clinical freedom "in its highest sense," since it removed the "fee barrier" both to medical advice and to the medicines doctors wanted to prescribe for their patients' "needs."

This Orwellian double-think conflicts with the events. As the state has footed the bill for drugs, appliances, etc., it has tried to control mounting expenditure by inspecting the books and penalizing "overprescribing." Such control must be arbitrary, as it is based on average prescribing and it undermines "clinical freedom" more than fees and poverty do. In prewar Britain doctors often charged little or nothing to poorer patients. It is now a Mad Hatter's teaparty: helping patients to pay by abolishing fees stimulates unrestrained prescribing—which government then must control by curbing clinical freedom.

Bevan did a "deal" with the doctors' leader who had advised him on consultants' salaries: he agreed to allow family doctors to earn fees from private patients and consultants to have private beds in state-owned hospitals. This "deal" illustrates the tactics of what Walter Lippmann called "gradual collectivism." The immediate task in 1946 was to entice family doctors and consultants into the state system, so capitation was retained and private beds conceded.

The doctors walked into the parlor. In 1976 a further stage in gradual collectivism was enacted by phasing out the private beds. In 1946 British doctors seemed to think that politicians were saints or immortals. (Some still do.) But the ultimate aim in 1946 was still a complete, comprehensive, "free" service. And it was being approached in 1976. The economic implication was finance by taxation. The political implication was state control. Bevan embodied in his legislation a "pledge" not to introduce a whole-time salaried service. Mrs. Castle later said "I and the government . . . are ready to renew in the legislation the pledge Nye gave that the right to private practice will be preserved." But not, in 1976, in state hospitals. And if private practice is isolated it will be easier to outlaw or banish (to Ireland? Europe?) as socially divisive and morally repugnant—two recurring descriptions in the political debate.

A politician's promise does not outlive him. Yet that is the promise British doctors accepted. There may be a fundamental lesson here for doctors everywhere, who are not (unsurprisingly) as skilled in politics as politicians. In state medicine around the world—in communist and developing countries both—doctors are subservient to politicians, who plausibly claim control over them in the name of "the people."

Bevan saw his tolerance of private ("pay") beds in National Health Service hospitals as an anomaly and a "defect" that mocked his principle of equal medical care free of price. Mrs. Castle tried to remove it.

THE YEARS BETWEEN

The stark contrast between the brave hopes of 1946 and the subdued puzzlement of 1976 reveals the real forces at work that propel centralized financing towards increasing control under the state if the system is to remain in being.

The government in 1976 would have liked doctors to forget the strains and stresses of the past thirty years and join with it in making state medicine work. In Mrs. Castle's words, it wanted them to help it find "a way of entering into a new, less bitter dialogue. . . . If the suspicions and resentments could only be broken down the profession . . . could play a great constructive part with government in . . . working out the right health priorities [etc., etc.]." And they could do this "not as civil servants, whole time conscripts or state slaves, but as free men fulfilling the ethic by which they seek to live."

This appeal reveals the intensifying political dilemma of centralized medicine. To continue in being it must have the assent of doctors; but to maintain the outward appearance of a system that can satisfy rising expectations it cannot tolerate the existence of health services for which patients pay because (they think) they are better. So the 4,500 private ("pay") beds in state hospitals, a mere 1 percent of the total 450,000, must be phased out. This displeases the senior hospital doctors at the very time they are asked to help the government run the system from which the beds they want are excluded.

The persecution of private medicine is to be pursued further. There have been hints that facilities such as X-ray for private patients are also to be excluded. If, exceptionally, they are used, charges are to cover their "full economic cost" (even though the patients have paid their taxes and social insurance contributions for them). Even private beds outside state hospitals are to be licensed on the credible ground of maintaining standards and protecting patients (a pretext for restriction used by the government in transportation). The number of these beds is not to exceed the number of beds phased out of state hospitals, so that whatever the public demand and the wishes of doctors, the private sector is to be prevented from growing. (On the other hand, Americans may be comforted to know that, like other foreigners, they will be allowed private beds denied to British nationals because of British demand for foreign exchange.)

As in education, the political tactic is to sharpen the gulf between government and private services, which can then be condemned as a preserve of the privileged. Government medicine is persistently described as "public," which conveys the flavor of Abraham Lincoln's "of . . . , by . . . , and for" the people. In practice the National Health Service is not "of" the people: there is no electoral machinery for the voter to indicate whether he is

for or against it. It is not run "by" the people but by harassed officials who marshal the patient more than they reflect his
wishes. And it cannot be "for" the people because 95 percent accept it with resignation that does not necessarily indicate
satisfaction.

But would the record of NHS in the years between 1946 and
1976 win the doctors' allegiance? Mrs. Castle conceded that it
was impossible to isolate the improvements in health that had
nothing to do with NHS—better diet, housing, environment.
Nevertheless she went on to some courageous claims.

First, NHS had produced "dramatic improvement" in health
care. New vaccines and treatments (many devised, of course, by
private pharmaceutical companies) had "totally transformed"
the effects of diphtheria, polio, whooping cough, measles, and
tuberculosis, which had all caused fewer deaths. How? Because
NHS had made them available to the poor as well as to the rich.
This claim is impossible to sustain unless there was no other
way to enable the poor to demand them. But the probability is
that Britain, the pioneer in state pensions and national health insurance, would have evolved other methods to help the poor
pay for medical care: perhaps income supplements or health
vouchers or state payment of premiums varying with income as
in Australia. But NHS had displaced them. The real "cost" of
NHS, which the advocates of state medicine avoid mentioning,
is the loss of more flexible methods of organizing and financing
medical services that would have been developed since 1946 in
its absence.

Second, said Mrs. Castle, there was only a small rise in the
proportion of the elderly registered as blind—largely because
cataracts had been diagnosed and treated early. This claim sup-
poses that the greatly improved living standards secured in the
intervening thirty years would—without the National Health
Service—have left people to continue stumbling about half
blind.

Third, improved ante- and postnatal care had greatly reduced
the risks of death in childbirth. This is just a careless example of

post hoc ergo propter hoc: in Europe there have been similar or even more marked improvements in such death rates and in infant mortality without universal "free" medicine. Fourth, "above all" the NHS had won "the deep seated loyalty of the vast majority of the people." This is a myth. There is no way of registering loyalty to the NHS except by showing individuals the costs of alternatives. When this was done for the Institute of Economic Affairs in 1963, 1965, and 1970, some 30 percent of a representative sample of all socioeconomic groups said they preferred to pay lower taxes and pay for health services by fees based on private insurance. This percentage would grow with the rising incomes.

Mrs. Castle summoned aid from a McKinsey Report, *Health Care—The Growing Dilemma*, from which she quoted the tepid conclusion that Britain "has achieved high overall health standards for a comparatively moderate slowly rising cost." It was a report commissioned by the 1970–1974 Conservative government which, in the pursuit of managerial efficiency, recommended administrative reforms that by almost common consent have done little more than inflate the nonmedical bureaucracy. It reshuffled the old cards in the hope that new tricks would fall out. Even before this reorganization the bureaucracy was growing. Between 1965 and 1975 total hospital staff grew by 28 percent from 628,000 to 803,000, but nonmedical administrative and clerical staff increased by 51 percent from 45,000 to 72,000. But during the same period the average number of beds occupied daily fell from 451,000 to 400,000. Another way of looking at it is that in 1965 there were 9.5 occupied beds to each nonmedical staff and in 1973 the number had fallen to 5.6. In 1965 two nurses coped with four beds; in 1973 they had only three beds but wards were nevertheless being closed "for lack of nurses," many of whom were caught up in nonnursing administration. These trends are characteristic of centralization.

But if NHS had achieved improvement, why the 1975–1976 crisis? Mrs. Castle failed to note that there had been a series of crises almost every five years since 1948. But she tried to explain that one. The National Health Service had not collapsed. It had continued to grow—to become the largest employer in the country, with more doctors, nurses, midwives, and health visitors than ever before. This is the familiar political and civil service reply to criticism. It invariably refers to quantity and almost never to quality. The increase in total numbers means very little without an analysis by kind, performance, quality, and—even more—a register of satisfaction by patients. But a monopoly has no way of discovering degrees of satisfaction. To say that 97 percent of the population has remained with the NHS means very little if there is nowhere else to go except at a higher additional cost. (NHS does not allow contracting out.)

Nevertheless, the 1975–1976 crisis had to be explained. The population was increasing; there were more people over seventy-five and their medical costs were growing. Far more people who had been rescued from killer diseases such as diphtheria survived to be crippled by disabling diseases such as arthritis. Growing medical knowledge yielded new treatments at higher costs. Medical labor costs had grown because of shorter hours. The new treatments were expensive. (One of Mrs. Castle's first decisions as minister was to introduce a "free" comprehensive family planning service.)

None of these would have caused recurring crises if the British people had been allowed to pay for medical care in the ways they preferred. Increasing population, technical knowledge, shorter hours, etc., were the common property of every major British industry, but they did not for those reasons suffer recurring crises. There must have been something else; and there was and is. NHS suffers from a chronic shortage of money because it is clumsily financed. It is financed by taxation which cuts the link between payment and benefit, not by the method that reveals (and indeed dramatizes) it—which is price or insurance premiums.

Between Mr. Bevan in 1946 and Mrs. Castle in 1976 came two other Labor ministers: Douglas Houghton in 1964–1967 and Richard Crossman in 1968–1970. It did not take them long to hit on what was wrong. And they said so plainly for all except the blind to see. In 1967 Houghton stated the problem precisely: "While people would be willing to pay for better health services for themselves, they may not be willing to pay more in taxes as a kind of insurance premium which may bear no relation to the services they receive." Crossman said it again in 1969: "People are prepared to subscribe more in a contribution for their own personal or family servity than they would ever be willing to pay taxation devoted to a wide variety of different purposes."

The lesson could hardly be made clearer. Price is a barrier to be surmounted, not a link to be snapped. Yet the myth lingers that the British yearn to spend more on NHS whether as individuals they can see the benefit or not—which they cannot if there is no price to which service can respond. A second myth is that the resulting smaller percentage of GNP spent on medical care than elsewhere (6 to 8 percent) does not matter—is indeed evidence of superiority—because NHS uses the resources it can raise more efficiently than the wasteful Americans, Canadians, Germans, French, and Australians use their larger resources.

This is the fatal flaw of all state systems: they spend *too little* on medical care. And the more health services are financed by taxes, the more debilitating becomes the weakness. The reason is that the greater the proportion of medical care financed by taxes, the more *private* benefits are financed by the method appropriate for *public* goods. That is the primary lesson that transcends international comparisons of mortality and morbidity.

Mrs. Castle's revelations were unintentionally revealing in this respect. For the fifteen years between 1948 and 1962 hardly any new hospitals were built and health centers were slow in starting (only one doctor in seven practices in them after thirty years); the reason, she concluded, is "the undemocratic nature of the structure which Nye set up." Competition for tax money is settled in a room in Number 10, Downing Street—the office of the Prime Minister. NHS, persisted Mrs. Castle, was lagging behind partly because "it has not been getting its fair share of national resources in recent years." Only a quarter of district hospitals were new since the war compared with a half of the schools and half of the houses. Why? Because education and housing are the province of local government and therefore are pushed by pressure groups, whereas hospitals are the province of appointed boards which are not so pushed. The solution, Mrs. Castle implied, was a more "democratic" structure of elected local government subject to pressure groups. Then doctors would have more hospitals, which they want. She did not add they would also have more political control, which they do not want. Where Mrs. Castle saw more "democracy," the doctors—rightly—see more party politics.

In a centralized system doctors are paid by the government, and new attitudes and habits in pay negotiation are soon learned. The "explosion of anger" over lagging income had ignited the new habit of striking, which had newly spread from doctors to nurses. The minister chided consultants who had learned the lesson of trade union "industrial" action and who demanded fixed hours of work and overtime pay. But it is the state system that changed them—and junior doctors and nurses—from professionals into clock-watchers. It is the confrontation with a single monopsonistic employer, the state, which can exploit its bargaining power and reduce medical incomes, that has changed the attitudes of doctors and nurses. From servicing patients, often imperfectly and with gaps and anomalies but steadily improving over the years, they have turned to hard bargaining with the boss.

"The real cause of the 1975–1976 malaise," said Mrs. Castle, was that "the most powerful men" in NHS had not been trained or conditioned to adjust themselves to new economic and social attitudes. "God and Mammon are at war in them." They were arguing—here at last Mrs. Castle approached the essence—that NHS was underfinanced and were "covertly" suggesting that health services financed solely by taxation would not satisfy the rising health expectations of a modern society.

Here, at last, the minister came to her Achilles heel. But she could not force herself to see it because "they [the doctors] are questioning the whole basis of Nye Bevan's dream." And that dream must not be disturbed. So she retorted not that the consultants' diagnosis was wrong, but that they had no alternative to NHS and its taxation. There were no large sources that could be tapped if the government allowed private money to pay a larger part in financing NHS. To probe and expose this "myth" was one reason for the Royal Commission.

Thirty years after NHS was established to remedy the defects, anomalies, injustices, gaps, and abuses of the old, gradually evolving, mixed system, it was still ordering enquiries into its own weaknesses.

THE CANADIAN EXPERIENCE

From its shorter experience with government financing in medicare, hospital insurance, and extended care (for people in nursing homes and homes for the aged), Canada broadly confirms the lessons of other countries. Despite some praise from administrators and academics in public health (who are sometimes apt to see all health services as public), the results of financing doctors and hospitals through government are uncommonly familiar. If resources for medicine are effectively decided by government, they are determined by the general condition of public finances and by party politics. Far from the long view, government tends to take the short view.

Government cost-sharing in Canada dates back to the early 1960s but experience of federal cost-sharing is only five to eight years old. A Royal Commission in 1964 was followed by the Federal Medical Care Act in 1966; but, primarily because of provincial anxieties about costs, the act did not take effect until 1968. Even then, only British Columbia and Saskatchewan joined; Alberta, Manitoba, Ontario, Nova Scotia, and Newfoundland waited until 1969 and Quebec, Prince Edward Island, and New Brunswick until 1971. Their participation followed pressure from the federal government (made effective by levying taxes in provinces that were slow to join). The following years saw hard bargaining between the federal and provincial governments. Medicine seems to have taken second place, as the patient has been seen not as a citizen requiring medical care but as a taxpayer perhaps willing to pay for medicine, whatever government could extract in taxes.

In June 1975 rising health costs, in part because government financing had hidden the costs of health services from the patient, forced the federal government to announce in the budget that it would restrict its contribution to cost-sharing in medicare and hospital insurance. This apparently high-handed decision, which the federal government could justify on grounds of budgetary stringency, has intensified the tension between the federal and provincial governments and made doctors feel themselves caught in a political maelstrom. Strong letters have passed between federal and provincial ministers of finance and ministers of health. Doctors have become increasingly doubtful about a system of financing that many accepted five years earlier. They see health services being squeezed between federal financial controls (limits, ceilings) and increasing demand from patients, rising costs, advancing techniques, and a growing population. The doctors complain theirs is the only salary group to be subjected to ceiling controls. Ontario has talked of cutting three hundred "active" beds and five thousand hospital staff; whatever the merits of this cutback, it makes good financial sense: the staff will be taken off the provincial payroll and put onto the federal unemployment fund (or welfare roll).

Governments short of finance tend to switch available resources from long-term investment to services used by voters in their daily lives. It now seems that medical research, new techniques and treatments, hospital laboratories and hospitals themselves will be kept short of funds (some made up by private effort). These government decisions are taken, as in all centralized financing systems, without reference to the preferences of individuals who may wish to continue health expenditures despite economic difficulties.

There are criticisms in Canada that patients use medical services excessively. This is another familiar result in other countries where financing is through government. It is easy to argue, as even such sophisticated observers as Professor Rashi Fein have done, that high charges deter patients and low charges are not worth collecting. But that does not destroy the case for pricing medical services. Charges and fees are the only source of information on costs that caution doctors against overprescribing and cause patients to think twice before taking the time and resources of doctors and hospitals that could be used for other patients. In the absence of charges, scarce resources must be rationed either by the providers, who may be competent to judge the efficacy of medicine but not its value to the patients who are given or denied it; or they must be rationed by government concerned with education, defense, inflation, preserving power, and much else; or they must be rationed by patients themselves, who will overdemand services with nil price. Public warnings to avoid calling doctors, as in the United Kingdom, are ineffective.

All systems are imperfect, but the least imperfect is a structure of varied charges that are not too high to deter patients nor too low to entice them to overuse medicine—that is, charges that minimize the deterrence and the overuse. Here again the limited experience of Canada reinforces that of other government systems of national health insurance or state medicine.

The central lesson of Canada, so far, is that patients should be kept very much part of the pay process by a wide variety of methods—deductibles, coinsurance, copayment, and others. These should be combined with assistance for low-income people so that they can join other patients as customers who pay—at least something but not too little—for what they want and who know the cost.

Canadian experience also suggests that, whatever the scope for capitation or salary, room should be found for direct fee paying, which is better than any other system in varying payment with the quality of service. The objection that patients are often not competent to judge quality in medicine is not conclusive. Neither are purchasers of other services sold by professionals with long training and refined skills in law, architecture, accountancy, and housebuilding. In medicine the patient does not have to be his own expert: he can use the family doctor as a medical broker to advise on the choice of specialist.

Government in Canada has largely replaced private insurance funds as the paymaster of doctors and hospitals. The method of insurance fund payment was not as good as direct payment by patients, but it is far better than payment by the sole agency of government. This way leads to the subjugation of the doctor, his clinical freedom, status, and income—as is evident in a wide range of national systems from the communist countries through Israel (payment by trade unions) to Belgium (insurance funds with strong bargaining power). From the ensuing confrontations the patient does not benefit.

Not least, Canada confirms that if medical care is centrally financed the tensions between overdemand by patients and arbitrary fluctuations from politicians' openhandedness (seeking votes) to overrestriction (fearful of inflating costs) gives patients the worst of all worlds. There is little comfort from Canada for the enthusiasts of national health financing or state medicine. It has not resolved the central dilemma: that the demand from citizens for underpriced or nil-priced medicine outruns the willingness to pay by taxes. The real task, in all countries, is to encourage people to see they can get better services by paying directly and to enable them to pay if they cannot because of low earnings or other obstacles. This system has its faults, but they can be dealt with more easily than the faults of capricious financing by governments. The Canadian federal government's precipitate restriction of cost-sharing is not an isolated act but a symptom of political control of medicine.

CONCLUSION: PRICE BARRIER OR LINK?

There are two principal lessons to be learned from other countries. First, the more centralized the financing of medical care, the more centralized and therefore standardized, conservative, and bureaucratic it tends to become. It is not an environment in which medical care thrives.

The second is that the faults of the variegated structures of health insurance, as developed in the United Kingdom before NHS and in recent years in the United States, are better remedied by working on the demand side than on the supply side. To remedy them by state medicine is to replace faults that can be remedied without violating the values of an open society by faults—rationing by queuing, resistance to change, overcentralization of decisions, political control—that have no remedies because they are organic elements in centralized political control of medicine.

The faults of voluntary or compulsory but still competitive insurance—gaps, uninsurable risks, duplication, "frills"—can be solved by methods that avoid the problems associated with centralized medicine: direction of (medical) labor, political control of medical schools, monopoly in state insurance, high taxation, bureaucracy, hectoring of patients ("Don't phone the doctor unless you must"), rationing by queuing, consolidation of bureaucratic vested interests, political confrontation with doctors (family, junior, hospital, or consultant), nurses, or administrators, extensive state ownership of hospitals and other physical assets, or generally increased state control over the *supply* of medical care. The faults can be treated substantially on the *demand* side by methods that aid development in the required direction: supplementation of low incomes (as in a reverse income tax, assistance with payment of premiums), deductibles (New Zealand and Europe), state insurance of catastrophic risks, information to suppliers and demanders, possibly standards. State services can then be more efficiently confined to environmental, preventive, and other "public goods," provision of beds and staff for long-term psychiatric and geriatric patients, though not in short-term general hospitals.

National health insurance fails in Western society because it cannot replace the missing link of price by ruthless rationing. Other Western countries—in Europe, in Australia—are trying to surmount the price barrier, and they are gradually succeeding in giving all their people access to rising standards of medical care. If the shortcut of snapping the price link succeeds, as it may for a time, it will be a Pyrrhic victory.

National health insurance and state medicine reflect the politician's earnest but erroneous belief that he knows better than the patient what to expect of the physician. Both patient and physician may wish to tell him: politician, heal thyself. But the record shows that he is incurable.

4

COTTON M. LINDSAY

ARTHUR SELDON

More Evidence on Britain and Canada

The negative effect on physicians of Canadian NHI. Geographical maldistribution of health care services. The cost of financing CNHI. The British free-for-all competition for medical care. A double cost to NHS consumers—taxes and rationing. Quantity replaces quality. Politics and the distribution of care.

Recent studies of both Great Britain and Canada provide new evidence of problems with centralized medical systems.

CANADIAN EVIDENCE

According to its supporters, the Canadian medical system has brought medical care within the reach of all Canadians by eliminating the price barrier. The reality, however, is very different. As we saw in the experience with the National Health Service (NHS) of Great Britain, lowering the price "barrier" does not extend access to care, since no new doctors are created to treat patients and no hospitals are financed or built. On the contrary, the apparent result of government medicine in the United Kingdom has been a net reduction of the resources channeled to health care. In Canada it is clear that national health insurance (NHI) has aggravated the geographical maldistribution of doctors and has made it more rather than less difficult for people in underdoctored areas to get care. And far from making care more accessible to low-income people, most of the funding for NHI has come from reduced spending for social welfare.

Declining Medical Resources

Canadian experience with government medicine has been shorter, and such trends are more difficult to identify. We note, however, that plans are already being implemented to reduce substantially the number of hospital beds in Canada, and real incomes of physicians have been severely eroded by a combination of government income controls and rapid inflation. At a time when real incomes of American physicians were rising, Canadian physicians experienced from 1971 to 1975 a decrease of 40 percent in their real incomes (Berger and Mosberg 1979, pp. 575–79). It is not surprising, therefore, that physicians are leaving Canada for the United States in record numbers (733 in 1977) and that many students attending Canadian medical schools do so with the explicit intention of practicing in the United States (Berger and Mosberg 1979, p. 577).

With such a drain on medical resources, it is clear that access is not being extended under Canadian national health insurance (CNHI). What has been the net distributional impact of its introduction? Results reported here are based on a recent study by Lindsay (1978) on the distributional impact of CNHI. We find that it has made health care *harder* to get for large numbers of Canadians, principally those living in already underdoctored areas, and that it has shifted a large portion of the cost of the nation's medical care onto the shoulders of the people with lower incomes.

Aggravating the Geographical Distribution

Although a few studies have reported that after CNHI adoption the poor began to consume a slightly larger share of the available medical care (Enterline et al. 1973, pp. 1174–78), Lindsay's results suggest that this is a short-term phenomenon. In the long run, the reimbursement system adopted by all provinces provides monetary incentive for physicians to spurn the ghettos and the hinterlands and to practice in urban environments already richly endowed with medical manpower. It matters little that there is no price barrier if there is no doctor. As a result of the reimbursement system adopted by CNHI, doctors are simply *moving away from the poor.*

The provincewide fee schedules adopted by CNHI eliminate compensating price differences, a part of the natural pattern of fees under a market system. A market pricing structure provides that physicians who practice in unattractive, poor, remote locations earn more than their colleagues who prefer to practice in attractive urban settings. When fees are equalized across entire provinces as under CNHI, the inducement to practice in less-attractive areas is eliminated. Fewer physicians will choose to practice in less-amenable communities since a particular service commands the same fee regardless of where it is delivered.

Evidence based on the numbers of physicians practicing in each county of each province over the decade from 1965 to 1975 was analyzed to determine whether this migration away from unattractive areas was taking place under CNHI. The number of physicians per capita was regressed on a number of variables measuring both demand and "attractiveness" of each county in various dimensions. This was done with data from 1965 and 1975 in order to provide a before and after view of location patterns for physicians.

The theory of medical pricing discussed above predicts that, once compensating price differences are eliminated, variables measuring location attractiveness will become more important in these equations. The predictions were borne out in the statistical results. The degree of urbanization, for example, was positively correlated with the physician/population ratio in 1965, indicating that it was regarded as attractive by doctors before CNHI. In the 1975 regressions, however, the importance of urbanization had doubled. Similarly, proximity to a medical school was found to be a positive feature in locational patterns in 1965. By 1975 the importance of urbanization had increased by 70 to 75 percent. In Quebec, for example, in spite of a general increase in the physician/population ratio of 33 percent over this decade, the ten least urban counties in Quebec experienced an increase in the physician population ratio of only 7.3 percent.

The Poor Are Paying for CNHI

The man in the street generally favors government free-for-all programs like national health insurance because he believes he is getting something for nothing. Since he pays little or nothing when he uses it, he gets the impression that it is "free." One of the most important lessons that economics teaches is that, while one person may get something for nothing (by taking it from someone else), it is simply impossible for *everyone* to have something for nothing. For each person who gets something for nothing there must be someone else who gets nothing for something.

Unlike American Medicare, which was explicitly financed by increases in the payroll tax, CNHI was introduced with no accompanying revenue measure. That no one *seems* to pay for CNHI does not indicate that it is costless—or that it costs less than it would if people paid it for themselves. In 1976 the budgetary cost of this program in Canada was $1,122 per family, and this does not include such items as dental care, outpatient drugs, home nursing care, eyeglasses, and hearing aids. The total economic cost of the program would also have to include the increase in queuing costs associated with reducing the money price. Economic theory suggests that lowered money prices will require some form of nonprice competition for medical care and, as we have suggested before, this often takes the form of longer queues for treatment. Evidence collected by Enterline (1973) supports this hypothesis.[1]

No Price—Lower Quality

Calculations of the cost of CNHI should also include consideration of its effect on the quality of care delivered. An important effect of reducing the price of care to zero is that the ensuing scramble for physician care puts doctors under pressure to hurry their patients through, to have their nurses and orderlies perform more tasks, and in general to reduce the quality of the care provided. Long lines in the waiting room and the lack of competition among physicians for patients will in the long run yield a product worth exactly what is paid for it.

The final result of this sort of indirect tax-financing is that it becomes extremely difficult to discover who is bearing all of these costs. The individual who calls for an appointment may realize that in some vague way his taxes are related to *total* spending on CNHI, but the exact way in which *individual* taxes and the full cornucopia of government give-aways are connected is only now beginning to be unraveled by economists.

If each government spending measure was accompanied by a tax bill which fully financed it, the task of identifying who was bearing what share of the cost would be much simplified. This is rarely done, however, and was not done at all in Canada when CNHI was adopted. Indeed, not only tax revenue but aggregate government spending over time do not seem to have risen by the full costs of these programs. This fact complicates our analysis further. If spending on health programs is not accompanied by corresponding expansions of the total budget, the conclusion seems inescapable that some older programs have been cut to finance CNHI. Part of the task of identifying who is bearing the cost of CNHI is therefore to find out which programs were cut and by how much.

This is not a simple task when incomes, tax revenues, and most government programs are growing. It requires predicting what the expenditure on each program would have been in the absence of CNHI, and then estimating the shortfall. These estimates were made econometrically with the following results: Roughly half of the Medical Care Act (MCA) program covering physician care was financed through budgetary expansion due to growing incomes and inflation. Some eight cents out of each dollar devoted to medical care came from *industrial* subsidies (largely the farm supports program). A similar amount came from diversion of funds which would otherwise have been spent on *police* and *protection*. The remaining program which was influenced by the introduction of the physician care part of CNHI was *social welfare* spending. Our regression analysis suggests that, for each dollar spent on CNHI, spending on social welfare was reduced by thirty cents.

The Hospital Insurance and Diagnostic Services Act (HIDS) provided government coverage of hospital services. It was introduced in the late 1950s, and thus predated the physician care part of the program by a decade. Our analysis indicates that this far more costly program was financed completely through diversion of funds from other programs, probably because the low rate of inflation during this earlier period produced no "fiscal bonus" in the form of increased taxes. We were able to identify two sources of diverted funds. Police and protection also suffered substantially under this program. For each dollar spent on HIDS, spending on police and protection was reduced by six cents. Due to the relative sizes of the two programs, however, this implied a significant impact on the latter. Our analysis indicates that a 10 percent increase in spending on HIDS (in the neighborhood of the mean) produced a 2.4 percent reduction in spending on police and protection. By far the most significant loser due to either MCA or HIDS, however, is social welfare. As noted above, the MCA program produced substantial diversions from social welfare. The diversions due to HIDS were larger, dollar for dollar, and because of the larger size of the HIDS program, even more significant on an absolute basis. For each dollar spent on the hospital insurance part of the CNHI we observed a seventy-one cent diversion from social welfare programs. A 10 percent increase in HIDS spending was estimated to produce a 9.5 percent reduction in social welfare spending.

Taken together, both parts of CNHI seem to have been financed largely through reductions in social welfare spending. Summing the MCA and HIDS coefficients, with appropriate weights for the relative sizes of the programs, indicates that roughly sixty cents out of every dollar spent on CNHI would otherwise have been spent on social welfare programs. Some analysis of the latter programs is obviously warranted. First, we can state categorically that the social welfare programs bearing the brunt of CNHI financing did *not* represent social financing of medical care which was phased out or administratively moved due to introduction of CNHI. Pains were taken to purge from these data any spending for health care under the category of social welfare. Our estimates thus cannot be dismissed as merely identifying an accounting shift which moved dollars spent on medical care from one program to another.

Most of the funds accounted for under social welfare spending (more than two-thirds) are "assistance to disabled, handicapped, unemployed and other needy persons." The remainder represents funds for workmen's compensation and family and youth allowances. It is the beneficiaries of these programs—the "underprivileged"—who have borne the burden of financing national health insurance in Canada. This is not to say that welfare spending has been cut in Canada since the introduction of CNHI. Welfare has grown—as have most other government programs—with growth in population, income, and inflation. But it has grown much less because of the new finance required for government health insurance.

Summary

In summary, then, Canadian national health insurance is not a "free lunch." It may superficially appear to have opened access to medical attention to all members of the public regardless of means. It has indeed reduced the money price of care to zero for Canadians, and in this sense the Canadian government has endorsed the notion heralded by Senator Kennedy that "health care is a right." The real implications of extending that right, however, are not what its authors and supporters intended. It has set in motion a relocation of physicians away from unattractive areas and patients (who, by the way, were already relatively underserved by physicians) toward urban and educational centers of the country. This result has almost completely neutralized, for rural and remote communities, the effect of the dramatic growth in the number of physicians in Canada over the past decade. It may spell severe deprivation for these areas in some future period when the nation is less well endowed with medical manpower.

Calling something a "right" may be thought by the naive to make it free. As this study illustrates, however, resources devoted to "public" (i.e., governmental) purposes must be diverted from private or other governmental uses. One disadvantage of shifting activities from the private to the "public" sector is that it obscures their total cost and, even more important, each individual's share of that cost. Only by complex econometric analysis was it possible to discover the distributional results of CNHI financing. In the name of extending the right to medical care to all, the rich as well as the poor, the Canadian government has shifted the burden of financing most of it onto the poor.

GREAT BRITAIN

The problems with the British National Health Service in practice are different but no less troubling. Although the British government has replaced the market in providing medical care, the fundamental functions of allocating resources to the various parts of the NHS remain to be performed. The principle burden of the British system is to improve on the market's resource allocation, but it is clear that in practice the British "nonsystem" has very little rationality in it at all (Lindsay 1979).

The problem is particularly evident in considering definitions of "medical need" which attempt to identify relative needs for care. Without money prices to restrict the allocation of scarce resources, the British NHS has substituted an illogical system of rationing by waiting time—so that some either drop out of queues or experience significant worsening of their conditions to such an extent that they become qualified for emergency treatment.

The problem of where to invest resources in new hospitals and the like, by the same token, has no relation to medical need. Instead, it is clear from the evidence that most decisions on capital investment for medicine in Britain are made for political rather than medical reasons.

Supply and Demand with No Prices

Ideally, government administration was to replace price rationing on the demand side with a more "sensible" system in which access to care was governed by "medical need" rather than by price. With the NHS, it was asserted, the economic barrier presented by price would no longer stand between the sick and necessary medical attention. But it is one thing to compose rhetoric about the goals of such a system and quite another to design and administer a system to achieve these goals. How does government organize a system which is to be responsive to medical need? Is it administratively possible to sift through lists of competing demanders to discover patients in gravest distress? These intriguing questions were never directly confronted by the architects of the NHS. They chose instead the usual government expedient of offering the medical care produced "free" to all. Rather than devising a *better* system for the rationing of medical care, they adopted the expedient of no "system" at all.

The results of such a "free-for-all" are well known to economists. As people may no longer compete for scarce resources with money, they compete in other ways. The most familiar nonprice rationing device is, of course, the queue in which access to the underpriced (i.e., "free") commodity is determined by willingness to wait in line. Such queues are extremely wasteful, resulting in the limit in a doubling of the cost of the "free" activity. British consumers pay for these services twice: once through taxation to pay for the resources required for production and a second time by devoting their own time (which may be more valuable than that of the doctor) to the queue in order to obtain it. Estimates of the magnitude of this social welfare loss associated with a hypothetical national health insurance plan for the United States are presented in Chapter 8. Those who question the importance or relevance of this analysis to government health care systems are invited to consider evidence on queues presented by the NHS.

Waiting is an ever-present feature of medical care under the NHS. Patients seeking the services of a family doctor may not always be able to make an appointment for that visit. They may have to appear at the physician's "surgery" (office) and wait in line. Even where there is on paper an effort to arrange appointments, patients have to wait. If more specialized talents are required, the patient must again wait for an appointment with the appropriate specialist. If the specialist determines that hospitalization is required, the patient is then put on a *waiting list* for hospital admission. Such prolonged, repeated waiting is unknown in any other Western country, but is not emphasized by the advocates of national health insurance in the United States.

Why Are They Waiting?

Waits for hospital admission are perhaps the most visible and politically troublesome aspect of this "free" system. The newspapers frequently cover stories of waits for surgery of six years and more; for hip replacements in a Midlands town it is four to five years. As hospital admission offers perhaps the best opportunity for the NHS administration to screen access on the basis of "medical need," it is instructive to analyze results of waiting list data for hospitalization.

There is little doubt that the NHS is effective in moving emergency cases into hospitals, but so is the American market-based system. Patients *in extremis* are usually treated promptly under both systems because it is the nature of hospital organization, and human nature on the part of doctors and nurses, to react with immediate attention to cases requiring it. It is not a unique merit of the NHS. The important question then concerns how care is allocated among those nonemergency cases of cold surgery or nonurgent treatment for whom relative "need" is more difficult to ascertain.

"Medical need" is therefore an ambiguous criterion. Although a panel of physicians might arrive at consensus on the relative importance of "needs" of various patients, no data exist on this criterion for cases treated by the NHS. It is thus impossible to test directly the importance of this consideration in the allocation of NHS resources. For this reason we decided to focus on the competing hypothesis that it was queuing that determined access to hospital care under the NHS. In his study, Lindsay (1979) reasoned that evidence supporting rationing by queuing would imply diminished scope for medical need or any other criteria in influencing access to NHS medical care.

Waiting for hospital admission is somewhat different from waiting for an office visit. Since time itself is valuable, time wasted in waiting rooms discourages some from joining the queue. The longer the wait, the more patients will be discouraged from seeking attention. Waiting in this case works like a price to discourage people unwilling to make this sacrifice of time to obtain service. Waiting for hospitalization requires no such cost to the patient. His name is simply added to a list and he goes about his business (if he is able) until his turn arrives.[2] This aspect of hospital waiting lists made necessary the development of a new theory of queuing in which queuing itself imposes no cost and does *not* therefore serve a rationing function.

Rationing by Delaying Treatment

The theory developed moved *delay* itself to the center of the analysis. It is not the *use* of time which discourages joining these queues; it is the *passage* of time which makes hospital care less attractive to some demanders and thus produces an equilibrium. Hospitalization for pneumonia is not very useful therapy if the expected delay for admission is five weeks. By that time the patient will have been treated by other (perhaps less effective) means. He will during this time either have recovered or become sufficiently worse so that he will have been admitted in emergency. The effect of this sort of rationing is thus to divert from hospitals cases which might be treated more effectively there, causing some in the process to deteriorate to the point at which more—and perhaps more intensive—hospitalization is required. Episodic cases will be "outwaited" by long-term cases even though the episodic may often represent more serious medical needs than the long-term. *This sort of rationing is therefore no less arbitrary than price rationing.*

Statistical tests by Lindsay to assess the validity of this reasoning strongly support the interpretation of the results of offering NHS hospital care free for all.[3]

Government Supply

Government "free-for-alls" thus evidently fail to ration care efficiently or equitably. Evidence of NHS performance in the organization of supply is perhaps even more discouraging. Few industries have ever been nationalized with louder ballyhoo than that which accompanied the introduction of the NHS. Its champions asserted that the "chaos" and "anarchy" which reigned before its adoption would yield to the rational orderliness of central planning and the genius of the British civil service. Early budgets were based on the assumption that disease would diminish or vanish once government had eliminated the backlog of illness produced by the imperfect allocations of the previous regime. High hopes and great expectations for the allocation of resources under government direction are usually disappointed. Results reported in the Lindsay study (1979) suggest that allocative experience with the NHS confirms this expectation.

Two rules govern success in government attempts to organize resource use. (1) Government planning is useful only to the extent that these plans conform to the political objectives of the party running the government. (2) Government direction of the production process is effective only to the extent that incentives of the bureaucrats making allocative decisions are consistent with achievement of the espoused goals. Analysis of NHS experience suggests that the system fails in both of these fundamental ways.

Government failure. Consider the organizational problem. Government administrators do not operate in a vacuum. They are just as concerned with job security and advancement as are employees of any private firm. Their behavior and performance in their jobs therefore depends essentially on their *perceived* or *measurable* success in the eyes of their superiors. Success for members of private firms can be gauged directly from the impact of their decisions on profits. Activities which increase efficiency and reduce cost will be rewarded. Activities which reduce cost at the expense of the *quality* of the product will be eschewed, since a deterioration in the product will be observed by customers and ultimately be reflected in sales and profits. It is a basic organizational weakness of government agencies that government administrators, when making allocative decisions, lack the discipline of maintaining quality (Lindsay 1976). This organizational failure is at least in part responsible for the frequently lamented preoccupation of government agencies with quantity rather than quality in their outputs.

This bias in favor of quantity against quality may be observed in at least three aspects of NHS performance. First, consider hospital capital investment. Table 1 presents capital expenditures per capita in real terms from 1950 to 1975. These figures document the frequently observed comment that the NHS, far from "rationalizing" hospital investment through central planning, merely nationalized existing hospital structure which predated it and then proceeded virtually to starve it of capital required for modernization and expansion.

The NHS bias toward lower-quality care may be observed, secondly, in data on hospital staffing. It would be predicted, according to the view outlined here, that government hospitals will overeconomize in the services they supply, that they would provide *less service* to patients than a more market-sensitive institution such as American proprietary hospitals operating in a competitive environment. This prediction is confirmed by data on personnel per bed in American proprietary and British NHS hospitals. Table 2 presents a comparison of these ratios from 1948 to 1975. Although staff per bed ratios in the United States exceeded those in the NHS hospitals in the opening years of the system, the difference in the figures has widened over the following thirty years. In 1950, for example, the staff/bed ratio

Table 1

Hospital Capital Investment per Capita in the United Kingdom and the United States* (various years)

Year	NHS	United States
1948		
1949		
1950	$1.26	
1951	1.20	$7.42
1952	1.20	7.29
1953	1.12	7.17
1954	1.04	7.05
1955	1.28	6.92
1956	1.23	5.76
1957	1.45	5.66
1958	1.80	5.56
1959	2.02	5.47
1960	1.97	5.39
1961	2.41	7.81
1962	2.89	4.37
1963	2.94	6.68
1964	4.44	9.75
1965	4.88	6.69
1966	5.22	5.03
1967	5.47	5.76
1968	5.40	7.16
1969		10.13
1970	4.97	7.39
1971	5.58	7.36
1972		12.57
1973		11.75
1974		11.35
1975		12.61
1976		

*Investment in both countries is shown in U.S. dollars (1970 = 1.00). U.K. data was converted, using prevailing exchange rates in each year.

89

in the United States exceeded that of the NHS by 40 percent. By 1960 this difference had grown to 47 percent, and by 1971 the excess of personnel in U.S. hospitals compared to the NHS had grown further to nearly 110 percent. Some part of this growth in U.S. spending on personnel may be attributed to the cost-plus hospital reimbursement policy adopted by the federal government for Medicare and Medicaid; the dramatic upward thrust in U.S. figures after 1965 is consistent with such an explanation. The entire difference cannot, however, be attributed to declining cost-consciousness on the part of U.S. hospitals associated with our own reimbursement practices. By 1965—that is, before Medicare and Medicaid—the difference in staff/bed ratios had reached 58.6 percent.

As a third example of the bias toward low-quality care under the NHS, consider the markets for physician care in the two countries. The *intention* of NHS administrators and the Review Body charged with setting pay for physicians was not, of course, to drive out of Britain highly qualified physicians and to replace them with lower-qualified (and less costly) physicians trained in Commonwealth countries; yet their pay policies have nevertheless clearly had this *effect*. Physicians and surgeons in Britain enjoyed a high standard of living before the adoption of the NHS. That standard has deteriorated steadily throughout the thirty years of association with government medicine. Table 3 presents calculations of rates of return earned by British general practitioners on the investment in their medical training. As calculations of rates of return earned on higher education in general range from 12 to 20 percent,[4] it is clear that doctors have been underpaid by the NHS. Even if we choose as the benchmark rate of return the lowest of these estimates (12 percent), we find that earnings of physicians in 1978 were too low by a factor of some 32 percent. Clearly, if the normal rate of return is toward the upper end of this range so that earnings received when doctors were brought into the system produced roughly a normal rate, they have been underpaid throughout the entire history of the NHS and the extent of underpayment cur-

Table 2
Total Staff per Available Hospital Bed in the United Kingdom and the United States
(various years)

Year	Total Personnel per Available Bed	
	NHS	United States
1948		.665
1949		.671
1950	.521	.727
1951	.524	.706
1952	.532	.716
1953	.539	.739
1954	.534	.790
1955	.534	.811
1956	.595	.855
1957	.606	.899
1958	.629	.932
1959	.647	.942
1960	.655	.964
1961	.674	1.016
1962	.697	1.044
1963	.702	1.099
1964	.710	1.113
1965	.723	1.146
1966	.745	1.254
1967	.761	1.318
1968	.756	1.388
1969	.758	1.470
1970	.767	1.570
1971	.793	1.664
1972		1.723
1973		1.804
1974		1.929
1975		2.062

Table 3

Rates of Return to Becoming a General Practitioner under the NHS in the United Kingdom 1948–1978

Year	Rate of Return
1948	22.6
1949	21.8
1950	20.6
1951	18.5
1952	18.8
1953	17.4
1954	15.9
1955	14.6
1956	13.4
1957	13.1
1958	13.3
1959	14.6
1960	13.3
1961	12.4
1962	12.3
1963	13.4
1964	12.0
1965	12.1
1966	12.3
1967	11.4
1968	13.9
1969	13.3
1970	13.5
1971	13.4
1972	12.2
1973	10.4
1974	9.2
1975	10.5
1976	8.7
1977	7.9
1978	6.5

rently is far larger than the 32 percent calculated on the basis of 12 percent.

Furthermore, the Lindsay study (1979) produced evidence that physician emigration from Great Britain is highly sensitive to changes in the rate of return earned on medicine. It was estimated that a 1 percent decrease in rates of return on medical training produces a 1.74 percent increase in the rate of emigration. In view of the extremely low rates of return calculated for the later 1970s, the outlook for emigration of doctors over the next few years may be a source of serious concern, especially to those who will lose their services—the British public.

Administrative failure.   In the final analysis, it is the second sort of failure listed above which is probably the source of the most serious and troublesome resource misallocation by government. The incentive structure within government organizations which fosters inefficiency in production might be altered and improved by one of several administrative changes. Monolithic agencies like the NHS might be broken up into competing suppliers of government-provided health care. Incentives might be devised to encourage competition in quality between government suppliers. But governments rarely adopt such management techniques, and the explanation lies in the nature of these organizations. Government organizations are first and foremost political institutions, not economic ones. Administrative changes that improve efficiency will be adopted only if economy is consistent with the political objectives of the people who have political power. One such pernicious conflict between efficient resource allocation and political objectives, with damaging consequences for health and democratic institutions, was analyzed in the Lindsay study (1979).

Geographical Maldistribution Continues: The Political Influence

A major improvement in the allocation of resources promised by the NHS was a more equitable geographical distribution of hospital resources. In that great philanthropic outpouring generated by the industrial era of the nineteenth century, the new rich built charity hospitals where they *appeared* to be needed: in places visited by these philanthropists. The West End of London, where most of these hospital builders lived, was the principal beneficiary, rather than the East End of London (which had the famous London-Teaching-Hospital and the charitable Jewish Hospital) and the industrial North, where many of the poor resided.

Twenty years after nationalization and government operation of these hospitals, little improvement in the geographical distribution of these resources was observed (Cooper and Culyer 1970). The Lindsay study (1979) sought an explanation for this failure by developing a model based on the supposition that the geographical distribution of spending between regions is influenced by their political importance rather than by efficiency or equity. The model was constructed around the following reasoning: the party in power will seek to extend its control over the government by spending a part of the budget to influence election results. Doing so involves a calculation by these politicians. They will not spend in districts they are certain to lose, for to do so would gain nothing. Nor will they spend in districts they are certain to win, because that also gains them nothing.

Politicians wishing to extend their power over government will spend money in districts likely to be politically precarious. It is here that votes influenced by government spending may deliver another party adherent to Congress—or in Britain, Parliament. A statistical model of the budgetary process was formulated which sought to explain variation in NHS capital spending on the basis of the anticipated closeness of individual races in forthcoming elections. This model was estimated in several forms using spending in each hospital region during six sample years in conjunction with three General Elections. The variable representing anticipated closeness in forthcoming elections was generally highly significant in these calculations. These robust results confirm beyond any reasonable doubt that *politics plays a role in the budgetary decisions of the NHS.*

NHS—the Contrast between Claims and Performance

In summary, the NHS performance has fallen short of the high expectations held for it at the time of its adoption in 1948 in both dimensions in which allocative systems must succeed. On the demand side, rationing by price has *not* given way to rationing of medical care on the basis of "medical need." Rather has it been replaced by rationing on the basis of duration of disease conditions. People with long-lasting conditions "outwait" patients whose demands for attention are short-lived. The NHS, whose queues for hospitalization seem to grow more outrageous every year,[5] has indeed created a "free-for-all" in this market. On the supply side, incentives within the Department of Health and Social Services (DHSS) organization have produced a system which sacrifices quality in the supply of health services at every turn. Less is devoted to capital and less to labor. Such resource stringency must worsen the quality of the final product. Furthermore, the resources which are devoted to health seek not efficiency in their allocation—that is, the optimum service to the patient—but rather the political consolidation of power by the politicians in control of government.

CONCLUSION

The most important lesson learned from these two systems is that eliminating explicit money prices does not eliminate the need for prices. Medical care, like all other scarce goods, must be rationed, if not by money prices, by some other way—by chance, queuing, or bribes. Eliminate the economic market and you give rise to a political market whose allocation decisions will surely be less rational than those of the economic market. The lessons in Britain and Canada should be borne in mind by those in this country who seek to emulate them.

5

COTTON M. LINDSAY

The Organization of Medical Care Markets

The dispute over economic efficiency and medical need. Allocation of medical care. Market mechanisms and nationalization. Externalities. The monopoly argument. Underproduction and overproduction of medical services. The relationship between physician and patient. Insurance and prepayment problems. The value of individual judgment.

One cause of the bitter disagreement concerning organization of the medical care industry is a lack of consensus on the *aims* of such organization. In most cases economic efficiency may seem a suitable objective for the allocation of resources, but another overriding concern is the matter of medical need. Too frequent and injudicious use of the word "need" by other social scientists has led economists to disparage arguments couched in these terms. What are needs, after all, but wants? And wants are the material of economics and efficiency. In certain cases, however, medical need has a different interpretation, an operational one, and economists should recognize and deal with this competing norm in resource allocation.

The statement that access to medical attention should depend on medical need has an undeniable validity in certain contexts. A doctor confronted by two patients, one in coronary arrest and the other with a bronchial inflammation, will invariably attempt to resuscitate the heart victim before attending to the other. Society would not tolerate an institution which fostered the alternative, regardless of the means of the two patients or their age or their political influence or any other test. Such examples come to mind when this statement is considered, and economists who refuse to admit the importance and singularity of these arguments toss their credibility to the winds.

The reluctance of economists to involve needs in their analyses has created a blind spot in the economic treatment of this allocative problem.[1] Because the issue itself is denied, the second—and ultimately the critical—question is never asked: Does the allocative issue posed in the above situation really shed light on the larger question of how medical care in general should be financed and organized? Both logical and empirical analyses suggest that it does not.

In the first place, allocation is an inadequate guide. There were roughly 35 million cases of heart disease in the United States in 1978 and only slightly more than one million deaths attributable to this cause. Thus there are fewer than ninety cases of heart disease for every doctor and less than three per doctor per year result in death. While other potentially lethal or crippling diseases are present in a modern society, of course, it is clear that our doctors, nurses, and hospitals would be wastefully underemployed if they were restricted to the care of those in obvious peril. A significant amount of medical attention is given to the relief of discomforting or disfiguring conditions which would otherwise cure themselves in time.

These facts have obvious implications for the question posed above. An allocative system responsive to needs alone must make difficult judgments as well as easy ones. We may all agree on the index of need required to make the allocative decision posed by critical cases and by trivial ones, yet most of the decisions will require the assessment and weighing of comparatively minor conditions which involve only the lowest level of mortal risk or impairment. What sort of allocative system best rations medical care on the basis of need for "difficult" decisions such as these? This is a problem which has attracted little concern, particularly in view of all the rhetoric devoted to the topic of needs and to their alleged implications for medical care systems.

One fact which is obvious, however, is that the device of merely offering all care "free" to everyone will not necessarily result in treatment of the neediest cases. If medical care is scarce relative to the amount sought and is not formally rationed by an explicit screening process, then queues will form and care will be distributed on the basis of the queuing process. When people must stand in line, care will go to those with little else to do. If people merely sign a list and wait their turn, care will go to those whose disabilities last the longest.[2] On the other hand, if medical care is sold, it goes to those willing to pay the most to obtain it.

None of these arrangements is likely to ration care in perfect correspondence to medical need. Certain members of society will gain special advantages from some methods while others will benefit from privileged access to another system. Indeed, it seems quite plausible that medical need is served equally by virtually any form of health organization. Few patients *in extremis* will be ignored under any system. Those who are so poor that they cannot purchase health care or insurance are not denied it today under our market-based system, nor have they ever been so far as I can determine. Today, of course, we have Medicaid not only for the poor but for the "medically indigent"—that bureaucratic euphemism for the irresponsible and improvident. Care for the poor and the improvident did not begin with this

program, however. It merely relieved states and local governments of a portion of the financial burden of caring for these patients. Long before governments took an active role in this area,
however, churches and charitable groups cared for the poor. I
have seen no evidence that their health or anyone else's is better
served now by our own or any other form of government
medicine.

Because of institutional features, Medicare and Medicaid have
resulted in increased spending for health care while arrangements such as the British National Health Service (NHS) result
in lowered expenditures per capita. Levels of spending do not
seem to be important to health, however. Statistical analysis of a
host of health indicators over the past sixty years fail to reflect
the impact of *any* government health initiative in Canada, Great
Britain, or the United States. When trend and intercountry
differences due to environmental, genetic, and economic factors
are controlled, we observe *no impact* on these indicators in the
years following adoption of National Health Insurance in
Canada, the NHS in Great Britain, or Medicare/Medicaid in the
United states (Lindsay 1979, Chapter2).

This is not to say, of course, that health organization makes
no difference. The fact that medical needs seem to be served
equally well under various systems merely heightens the importance of other criteria. If medical needs are taken care of "in-
framarginally," then the balance of health care should be allocated according to the standards governing resource use in other
consumption activity, i.e., economic efficiency.

MARKETS AND HEALTH CARE
ORGANIZATION

The production of most goods and services is left to markets, at
least in Western countries, and with good reason. It is widely
acknowledged that market organization will produce, if not the
optimum allocative results in many industries, at least tolerably

good results—better in most instances than could be expected of nationalized industries. Markets, to a greater or lesser degree, reward the movement of resources from areas and applications where they are abundant and less valuable to those where they are scarce and more valuable. They reward the introduction of cost-reducing technology. These results are generally salutary.

This is not to say that there exists among policymakers or economists a broad consensus that markets are invariably preferred for the organization of economic activity. For many activities market solutions are rejected on the grounds of efficiency. Lack of central direction is no longer treated as adequate evidence for the desirability of central direction; such direction is nevertheless frequently prescribed in cases where markets are alleged (with varying degrees of plausibility) to fail. The "sophisticated" efficiency arguments for government involvement in medical care today seek to identify in medical markets one or another of the recognized causes of market failure.

One cannot therefore consider the desirability of this type of government intervention in the health care industry without reference to the consequences predicted by those who see such problems to be rife. We shall devote the balance of this chapter to a discussion of these potential efficiency problems associated with the provision of medical care.

Externalities

Apart from monopoly, externalities (as they are conventionally styled) represent the oldest recognized form of market failure. These are alleged to arise when the price of an activity fails to reflect either its full social value at the margin or its full social cost. Should the market be characterized by the former type of externality, the activity will be underproduced. Overproduction results in the second case. The conventional solution is to subsidize those which are underproduced and tax those which exhibit the opposite problem. Medical care is more often associated with the "demand failure"—underproduction.

Although externality analysis is widely discussed in connection with many policies, its limitations for guiding concrete policy decisions are crippling. If market values fail to reflect the marginal social value of activities, where is one to find alternative measures? If the value placed by a patient on treatment of his respiratory infection is less than society's value of that treatment, then what is the magnitude of the implied subsidy? As health care consumption is already heavily subsidized even in countries like the United States where its organization remains in the market sector,[3] does the alleged presence of externalities imply even larger subsidies or are they presently adequate or excessive?

Furthermore, externalities—should it be decided that present subsidies are inadequate—imply no further intervention than an extension of policies already practiced by various levels of government in America. They imply at most an extension of aid to medical and nursing schools and to students and more financing for hospitals. Nothing in this doctrine supports nationalization of the health insurance industry.

Monopoly

A copious and influential literature dating from the mid-1930s maintains that the tightly regulated and licensed professional structure of medicine has produced "barriers to entry" in this profession. Rather than protecting the interests of consumers, these regulatory agencies have been "captured" by the profession, according to this scenario, and used to control entry into medicine and to prevent "price cutting" by existing practitioners (see Friedman and Kuznets 1945; Kessel 1970; Rayack 1967). It might be argued that a centralized reimbursement system which negotiated directly with professional organizations over fees would have the bargaining power to overcome such cartels.

This argument is difficult to credit on two grounds. First, serious methodological questions have been raised concerning interpretation of the original evidence adduced to support the entry barrier hypothesis. What appear to be monopoly earnings of physicians in the earlier studies are revealed under more careful scrutiny to be competitive (see Lewis 1963; Lindsay 1973). Detailed examination of the behavior of licensure bodies and medical schools—the alleged instruments of such a conspiracy—also fails to support the monopoly argument (see Leffler 1978; Lindsay and Hall 1980). There is serious disagreement, in other words, in regard to the presence of such a market failure in the U.S. medical industry.

Secondly, and perhaps more to the point of the present work, there is also doubt concerning the nationalized "solution" to this problem. Whatever barriers to entry into medicine are actually present have existed there for many decades under the supposedly watchful eye of government. Stigler (1974) and Peltzman (1976) have repeatedly indicated that agencies introduced by government to confront large and concentrated economic interests in the private sector are typically "captured" by these interests and used to consolidate cartel power.[4] We have no reason to suspect that boards empaneled to set fees for doctors will not be similarly infiltrated. If recent government dealings with public employee groups are indicative of what we can expect from these negotiations with the medical profession, little relief from any alleged cartel is in store.

Moral Hazard

While externality analysis and the possibility of monopoly are leading one set of critics to the conclusion that health care is underproduced by markets, the hypothesized presence of moral hazard leads another to the conclusion that markets overproduce care. Moral hazard is an insurance-based phenomenon. When an activity is insured, its price is lowered to the demander. The effect is similar to an externality in the sense that people will tend to consume insured services beyond the point at which social value is equal to social cost.

Unlike externalities, however, the extent of moral hazard can and has been measured. Martin Feldstein (1973) has estimated that an increase in health insurance deductibles which doubled the average copaying rate (from 33 to 67 percent) for the U.S. market as a whole would produce net welfare gains in the neighborhood of $4 billion yearly. The central problem here is that "excessive" resources may be attracted to the health industry by virtue of the fact that insured demanders are not (individually) bearing the full cost of the services they use. It might be argued, therefore, that a system in which supply is made unresponsive to demanders would not fall victim to moral hazard.

Agency Relations

The problem of moral hazard is made more severe by another alleged market failure, the so-called "agency relationship" which can exist between physician and patient. Agency describes a relationship in which the supplier provides to the demander both a service and advice concerning the demander's need for the service. Within limits—and what determines these limits is the weakest part of this theoretical development in its current state—providers function as both suppliers and demanders in such markets. Under these circumstances it is possible for unscrupulous doctors to take advantage of such a situation to prescribe more of their service than patients would buy if they knew what they were really getting. This problem is compounded by the presence of insurance. Such an arrangement combines the consumers' indifference to costs at the margin with the physician's perverse economic incentive to overprescribe care.[5]

It is important to recognize that these implications stand in contradiction to those discussed earlier. Nationalization was suggested in that discussion because market organization produced too little care as indicated by patients' "needs" in the one case or allocative efficiency in the other. Externality analysis and monopoly both imply that output will be suboptimal.

Here the market failures of moral hazard and agency supply combine to produce the opposite result. Nationalization is advanced as a solution to these problems because it severs the connection between market demand (at a zero price) and resource allocation preventing *excessive* investment in health care. Let us consider some evidence on people's revealed preferences for such a solution, however. The problems of moral hazard and agency supply are greatly reduced by a shift of financing from fee-for-service to prepayment. If providers are no longer reimbursed for additional units of service prescribed, then the incentive for them to prescribe excessive service is eliminated. Indeed, a switch to prepayment may produce incentives which overcompensate, but that is not really important here. The point is that a market alternative to the present regime is available which does not contain the adverse incentives just discussed.

Prepayment organization has in fact been a feature of the American health care landscape for many years. Certain groups such as HIP of New York and Kaiser-Permanente of California have been very successful at offering medical insurance packages containing provider prepayment features. Generous subsidies were made available by the U.S. government to groups forming to offer such packages through the Health Maintenance Organization (HMO) Act in 1973. Yet few people elect to insure in this way. In 1977 only about 6 million Americans had medical insurance with an HMO. This is less than 3 percent of the total health insurance market.

NATIONALIZATION V. MARKETS

Part of the reluctance to embrace the HMO concept, as Enthoven argues in Chapter 10, is undoubtedly due to the fact that the savings implicit in these plans are often not passed on to the individual subscribers. Allowing them to keep such savings and thereby encourage fair competition between the two approaches is an important reform which is long overdue. At the same time, even where fair competition exists between prepaid and fee-for-service plans, many people are willing to absorb the higher premium cost associated with fee for service to obtain the personalized service and other perceived advantages of this traditional delivery mode. And this is true even though at least part of that higher premium results from problems discussed above. If people will pay this higher cost, does it not suggest that the shortcomings they see in HMOs will be present in spades with nationalized health care? In other words, is it not possible that consumers may prefer market-based health care with all its warts to a nationalized system? Moreover, it's easier to get into a nationalized system than it is to get out.

6

DAVID A. STOCKMAN

W. PHILIP GRAMM

The Administration's Case for Hospital Cost Containment

The call for "command and control" regulation of health care costs. Opposition to the Hospital Cost Containment Act. Intensity growth and its effect on hospital prices. Personnel, specialized facilities, and malpractice. Increased outpatient services. "Waste substitution." Mandatory revenue controls.

When viewed with the benefit of hindsight, the 96th Congress will be seen as a watershed period in the development of federal health policy. The focus for this policy redirection is the Carter

107

administration's Hospital Cost Containment Act, introduced in both 1977 and 1979 as the proposed solution to the problem of rapidly rising system costs. Even those, such as Senator Kennedy, who are committed to further additions to the rapid surge in demand that was generating cost problems in the first instance, became convinced during this time that only stringent "command and control" regulation of the public utility variety could save the nation from the spectre of health care as a luxury affordable only by the few.

Dramatic action was called for. Hence the call went forth from the Carter White House to every part of the land signaling holy war for the bill's enactment. The Congress was assured that this legislation was the "single most important thing" that they could do to combat double-digit inflation. Armies of senior citizens were unleashed to lobby the Congress on behalf of this crucial legislation. And the disbursement of federal funds under the president's discretion soon evinced a pattern explainable only in light of the vote counts in the key committees of the House of Representatives through which the administration's bill sailed.

Given this all-out onslaught, it seemed impossible to most experienced observers that the regulatory armada could possibly founder on the rocks. Yet founder it did, crashing to shore upon an overwhelming wave of opposition to the revenue control provisions of the president's legislation in the key House vote.

In the wake of this vote, many concluded sadly that the Congress simply lacked the resolve to tackle the troubled but politically sacrosanct health care industry. We suggest, however, that the reality is in fact far different. For the scuttling of the Hospital Cost Containment Act, far from being a dismal legislative breakdown, was rather a huge political success that may well prove to turn the tide against the confused thinking, muddled platitudes, and downright bad logic that have dominated federal health care policy since the 1960s.

The case advanced for the revenue limits that formed the core of the administration's proposal is premised on the grounds that the hospital industry is in the grip of a mysterious hyperinflation induced by endemic flaws in the market structure of the health care sector. Normal market forces fail to function, it is argued, because physicians exert undue control over the volume of services ordered and hospitals compete for physicians with glittering high-technology toys rather than for patients on the basis of price. Given the complete absence of cost-consciousness in the system, the conventional wisdom holds, only regulatory surrogates for the normal market incentives—centralized facilities planning, utilization reviews, and outright revenue controls—have any hope of rationalizing the operation of this $200 billion industry.

The empirical evidence on system overcapacity—and the astonishing increase in aggregate expenditures—lend a certain surface plausibility to this notion. Yet when examined in more detail, it soon becomes clear that excessive capacity and costs are not inherent characteristics of hospital markets but are rather predictable consequences of the massive federal effort of the 1960s and 1970s to pump up demand for health services. In fact, it would be astonishing if the health care industry *had not* responded to the incentives produced by virtually unlimited demand for more and better services.

The fatal error of the Carter administration in presenting its case for a regulatory solution lay in its attempt to sidestep this underlying issue of excess demand for health services by concentrating single-mindedly on aggregate indices of cost problems in the industry. For once a majority of the members of the Congress stumbled through this smoke screen it became quite clear that the administration was pressing for a considerable grant of regulatory authority over the day-to-day operations of the hospital industry almost without regard to the consequences for the future development of the industry. Once the initial confusion of sorting fact and fancy from the blizzard of statistics produced by the Department of Health, Education, and Welfare (HEW) had been eliminated, a majority of the House became convinced that the problem was far too fundamental and complex for the proposed regulatory quick-fix to be anything but an engine of chaos in the nation's hospitals.

DRAMATIC GROWTH IN INTENSITY OF HOSPITAL SERVICES

One major confusion results from the inadequacy of conventional hospital price measures. Neither the consumer price index (CPI) daily room and board rate index nor the "expenses per case" data published by the industry and HEW account for quality improvement. This contrasts sharply with other major items in the consumer price index—such as automobiles and consumer appliances—where the Bureau of Labor Statistics makes periodic downward adjustments to account for quality improvements. Yet quality improvement has been the principal outcome of the tremendous increase in demand for hospital services through third-party payment.

An accurate measure of the true rate of hospital price change must allow for expanded quantity and quality of actual services. Economists have attempted in recent years to quantify the breakdown between the two primary components of hospital cost increases: several inflation factors, and increases in the quantity and quality of *inputs* in the typical bundle of services provided per patient day or per admission.[1] While the task is complex, the Health Care Financing Administration has concluded that nearly 40 percent of the average increase in hospital expenses during the last decade is accounted for by improvements in quality (see Table 1).

The sudden dip in the rate of intensity growth during the 1971–1974 Economic Stabilization Program controls is particularly interesting. Unable to substantially reduce inflation in labor and supplies purchased, to stay within the mandatory charge increase limits hospitals were forced to restrict severely the increases in their service capabilities. In 1974 controls were

TABLE 1   Intensity and Inflation Components
of Hospital Price Change*

	1969	1970	1971	1972	1973	1974	1975	1976	1977	1978
Inflation	6.2%	7.8%	6.4%	4.4%	5.2%	10.0%	13.5%	5.8%	7.3%	7.5%
Intensity increases	7.5	6.4	5.1	7.6	3.1	1.2	4.2	8.0	6.4	4.2
Total	13.7%	14.2%	11.5%	12.0%	8.3%	11.2%	17.7%	13.8%	13.7%	11.7%

Source: Deborah L. Allen, "HCFA Non-Labor Factor Price Increase Index for Hospitals," unpublished ms., 1977. American Hospital Association, *Hospital Statistics, 1978.*
*Hospital prices measured as expenses per case.

released from most sectors of the economy, but the administration sought to retain hospitals within the Phase IV limits then proposed. As a result, hospitals faced an enormous surge of supply-cost inflation that further inhibited intensity increase well into 1975. The subsequent dramatic catch-up in hospital growth rates, as we have seen, was a direct result of these controls.

The issue at stake in any effort to restrain the trend rate of growth in hospital expenditures, then, is the rate of intensity growth. Single-sector regulatory initiatives in the hospital field, because they are unable to cope with price movements in uncontrolled input factors, can only be focused on moderating the trend rate of intensity growth.

Any such effort, however, inevitably involves a sharp confrontation between the desire to contain costs and the desire — explicit in current federal health policy —to support continued improvements in the access of the American people to quality health care. To the extent that intensity increases in hospitals are the *essential element* in hospital service improvements, slashing quality improvements in the name of controlling costs will always be a counterproductive endeavor.

The case has been advanced, of course, that the lion's share of hospital intensity increases are in fact inherently wasteful; that the most recent intensity increases involved unnecessary expenditures for superfluous gadgetry, massive X-ray overdoses, and unneeded hospital beds. It has also been argued that these intensity improvements have little effect on the health of the American public. Indeed, former HEW Secretary Califano recently suggested that cutting such intensity increases will actually *improve* the health care system. According to Mr. Califano, the excessive usage of low-level radiation and deaths due to unnecessary surgery have made our health care system a *very dangerous place* from which the public should be protected whenever possible.

The fact, however, is that improved hospital services have had a readily demonstrable impact on treatment results and health status of Americans. To be sure, health care is not the only contributor to health status; equally important are such factors as diet, exercise, and environmental conditions. But some recent health improvement is properly attributable to improved hospital care. For instance, in the decade between 1965 and 1975 the heart disease death rate per 100,000 population in the most vulnerable category (aged forty-five to fifty-four) fell by 21 percent—undoubtedly reflecting both improved treatment and better health and dietary practices.

In other areas it is possible to isolate health improvements that directly reflect improved quality of hospital care. Between 1965 and 1975, for example, infant deaths within seven days of birth—the period after birth most closely tied to postnatal services in hospitals—fell from 15.9 per 1,000 births to 10.0, or by 37 percent. Similarly, deaths from accidents fell from 25.4/ 100,000 to 17.2/100,000 because of improved emergency treatment. And the in-hospital death rate for heart attack victims has declined by 30 percent as a result of the diffusion of coronary intensive-care units.

This evidence suggests that arbitrary restraints on further quantity improvements could seriously retard further improvements to health care, particularly for those now medically underserved.

THE ANATOMY OF INTENSITY

In the myriad recent changes in the hospital service package, four main areas, taken together, have generated the 5–6 percent annual service improvements: changing personnel mix, improved diagnostic methods and equipment, improved treatment methods and facilities, and the changing mix of patients that hospitals serve.

Personnel—Changes in Quantity and Quality

Personnel costs have increased rapidly in this decade for three basic reasons: the growth of specialized services, the increasing paraprofessionalization of many aspects of medical care, and the general administrative workload associated with increasing service complexity and government regulation (see Table 2). These increases have a particularly significant impact on the cost of hospital services, since personnel generally accounts for at least 55 percent of the average hospital budget.

In addition to increasing *numbers* of persons involved in the delivery of care to each patient, personnel quality has also improved. This is particularly apparent in the nursing profession, in which a significant—and increasing—percentage of highly trained nurses are providing services in hospitals. In 1968 only 22.7 percent of all advanced nursing students were studying advanced clinical practice; today the figure exceeds 60 percent. As a result, nearly 8 percent of today's active nursing force have formal degrees beyond LPN (Licensed Practical Nurse) or RN (Registered Nurse) certificates.

Increasingly specialized personnel training is also required for operation of increasingly technology-intensive services. As hospitals bid for trained personnel, the growing demand is reflected in rapidly rising wage rates. Thus while wage rates for emergency room personnel have risen 36 percent over the last six years, average wage rates for persons in sophisticated areas of medical technology—intensive care units, radiology services, and surgical recovery facilities—rose 45–55 percent. These trends are likely to continue, despite the gradual slowing of the tendency toward greater capital expenditures by hospitals.

Increasing Diagnostic Services

A second major contributor to improvements in hospital services has been the growth in volume—and in quality—of hospital diagnostic procedures (see Table 3).

Not all of the factors shown produce disproportionate increases in hospital costs. During the period shown above, for example, the volume of laboratory tests rose 60 percent but their average unit price rose only 18 percent—far below the general inflation rate. The change is largely due to mechanization of large-volume standard tests in medium and large hospitals.[2]

Considerable controversy has centered on the costs of increased diagnostic testing. In most other industries, new technology and procedures are introduced only to reduce net unit costs. Yet intensity increases in health care have often increased the costs.

A classic example of the problems associated with understanding the impact of diagnostic technology on the practice of medicine is the case of the much-maligned Computed Axial Tomography (CT) scanner, a technological breakthrough that has added considerably to diagnostic capabilities. The CT scanner operates by building up a cross-sectional picture of various areas of the head and body and displaying it on a screen or printing it on paper. Armed with these detailed "photographs" of the interior of the body, physicians, without having to resort to exploratory surgery, can get a considerably better reading on ab-

TABLE 2   Man-Hours per Admission for
Various Personnel Groups
1971–1976

Category	1971	1976	Increase Hours	Increase Percent
Doctors/dentists	2.8	3.4	.6	21.4
Residents/interns	3.5	4.1	.6	17.1
Other trainees	2.2	2.7	.5	22.7
Registered nurse	23.8	29.2	5.4	22.7
Practical nurse	12.2	13.2	1.0	8.2
Other	103.8	116.2	12.4	11.9
Total	148.3	168.8	20.5	13.8

Source: American Hospital Association, *Annual Survey.*

TABLE 3   Common Hospital Procedures Performed
per 100 Admissions

Procedure	1971	1976	Percent Change
Blood units drawn	14.1	15.9	12.8
Diagnostic X-rays	152.8	191.7	25.5
Laboratory tests	1,561.3	2,496.1	60.0
Nuclear medicine procedures	11.7	22.1	89.7

Source: "Hospitals," *Journal of American Hospital Association* (August 1976).

normalities in each body segment than that obtained by the limited results of X-rays. The result can be significantly improved diagnosis at a *much lowered cost* than would be available under traditional methods. Table 4 compares the relative cost of using the CT scanner with the cost of using traditional diagnostic methods in diagnosing three illnesses.

Once in place, of course, these diagnostic machines may not always be used for the most cost-effective reasons. While capital costs can be amortized over more and more units of testing as utilization rises, the high variable costs of labor and supplies must be added to each scan. As a result some physicians will order questionably necessary (this does not mean undesirable) use of the CT scanner, particularly for the more expensive total body scans. It does *not* follow, however, that all such scans so ordered do not improve diagnosis or that a hospital's possession of a scanner is always questionable. These questions can only be settled through case-by-case reviews.

Defense against Malpractice Suits

Another controversy centers on the extent to which physicians increase testing to combat the threat of malpractice suits. Estimates of the annual costs of such "defensive medicine" range from $1 billion to $6 billion annually. A significant number of malpractice cases have involved negligent failure to perform tests or procedures that might have prevented subsequent death or disability.

Federal health policy mandarins continually deplore this practice of defensive medicine. Apparently they believe that it produces costs out of proportion to any health benefit received by the patient. Nevertheless, short of completely restructuring the malpractice liability laws of fifty states, physicians have essentially two options: test or be sued. So test they do. Of course, even physicians who are generally critical of the level of defen-

TABLE 4   CT Scanning versus Conventional Diagnosis Comparison of Total Costs

Diagnostic Category	Avg. Days to Final Diagnosis	Average Stay	Estimated Costs			
			Tests	Room/ Board	Exploratory Surgery	Total
Abdominal mass:						
Conventional	9	17	$885	$2,261	$1,800	$4,946
CT	3	11	445	1,463	0	1,908
CT savings	6	6	$440	$ 798	$1,800	$3,038
Obstructive jaundice:						
Conventional	10	25	$448	$3,325	$ 0	$3,773
CT	4	19	154	2,527	0	2,681
CT savings	6	6	$294	$ 798	$ 0	$1,092
Pelvic mass:						
Conventional	9	28	$732	$3,724	$1,800	$6,256
CT	2	21	597	2,793	0	3,390
CT savings	7	7	$135	$ 931	$1,800	$2,866

Source: *EMT Clinical Research* (May 1977).

117

sive medicine practiced by their colleagues nevertheless concede that an extensive diagnostic work-up, while not always indicated by obvious symptoms, will often improve diagnosis, speed treatment, and lower its cost.

In summary, while lab testing has certainly been on the rise and may well have been substantially increased by the influence of malpractice, to conclusively demonstrate that this rise has been with or without net benefits is outside the scope of the activities proposed by regulatory solutions focused on revenue aggregates. Indeed, such regulation contains a built-in prescription for unproductive conflict. The cost containment ceilings bear down on hospital charges for ancillary source billings such as lab tests, but in the real world of hospital practice the frequency and extent of such tests are almost totally within the control of individual physicians. In the absence of fundamental change in the malpractice liability climate, there is no reason, *a priori*, to believe that hospitals will be successful in reducing test utilization rates. Nevertheless, they will be liable for the resulting costs.

The Diffusion of Specialized Facilities

Nothing demonstrates the impact of changing technology and procedure in the practice of medicine within hospitals better than the diffusion of specialized hospital units. This diffusion in the last decade has been due partly to the expanded use of existing facilities and partly to the expanded number of hospitals equipped to perform various tests and procedures (see Table 5).

These new facilities are considerably more expensive to construct—and to operate—than the general medical/surgical capacity of the hospital. For example, while the cost of the average hospitalization for surgery runs in the range of $1,500 for hospital costs, the average hospitalization for open-heart surgery can cost close to $10,000. Similarly, hospital charges for stays in a burn unit can run three to four times the average medical/surgical bed rate. The reason for the considerable cost of

TABLE 5 **Percentage of Community Hospitals with Selected Specialized Facilities 1965–1978**

Facility	1965	1978	Percent Change
Cardiac intensive care	0.05%	31.7%	N/A
Burn unit	0.05	2.8	N/A
Mixed intensive care	26.7	67.7	154%
Occupational therapy	11.2	22.1	97
Home care department	5.0	9.5	90
Pharmacy services	58.5	91.4	56
Physical therapy	51.7	80.6	56
Cobalt therapy	10.5	14.6	39
Blood bank	61.4	71.8	17

Source: American Hospital Association, *Annual Survey.*

these new treatment modalitics is twofold: specialized units generally require considerably higher personnel intensity, and capital costs to construct and equip them are higher.

Aggregate national statistics, of course, do not indicate the wide variations among regions in the diffusion of such hospital facilities. For example, while the national average shows 32 percent of all hospitals in the nation having cardiac intensive-care units, the actual data range from 16 percent in New Hampshire to 55 percent in the District of Columbia. Similarly, 81 percent of all Rhode Island hospitals have blood banks, yet only 37 percent of Wyoming hospitals are equipped with their own in-house blood bank facilities.

The argument has been made that these specialized facilities have been diffused too widely. But regional disparities point out the difficulty of establishing numerical quotas for specialized hospital facilities on the basis of population alone. On a national-average basis, for example, there is roughly one burn-care unit per 1.4 million population. When one considers that the entire State of Alaska has a population of only 405,000 people, however, it is another thing to consider where such facilities should be geographically distributed. To say that installation of a burn unit in an Alaskan hospital would give it 3.5 times the needed capacity, based on national averages, would be to completely miss the point.

AS CASES GET HARDER, COSTS GO UP

Part of this relentless rise in the intensity of hospital staff, equipment, and procedures is directed at the population as a whole, but a significant portion of these increases is due to the fact that the hospital's "customer" is changing over the years. Even if hospitals did not increase the capacity level of staff and facilities over time, costs would still rise significantly above the inflation rate. There are two basic reasons for this: the tremendous growth of outpatient services, which are gradually emptying hospitals of easy, low-cost cases, and the general aging of the population.

It goes without saying that the actual cost of treating patients in hospitals varies from case to case. As noted above, the average cost of admitting and treating a heart patient is several orders of magnitude greater than the cost of a short hospitalization for the routine removal of a cyst. For this reason, a gradual change in a hospital's patient-case mix toward more difficult cases tends to drive up its average cost per admission faster than even the increases in costs of normal inflation and average service intensity. There is compelling evidence that, on average, hospitals are treating more difficult cases today than they were just ten years ago. Moreover, this trend toward more difficult cases will continue, and may even accelerate, over the next thirty years.

Part of the reason why hospitals are taking on more difficult cases is an express federal policy favoring treatment of "the easy ones" on an outpatient basis. The evidence shows that hospitals

TABLE 6 Outpatient Visits to Community Hospitals
1965–1977

Year	Outpatient Visits (millions)	Inpatient Admissions	Outpatient Percentage of Total Hospital Expenditures
1965	92.6	26.4	9.2%
1966	106.5	26.9	9.1
1967	109.9	27.0	8.8
1968	114.1	27.3	9.4
1969	120.8	28.3	8.7
1970	133.5	29.3	9.1
1971	148.4	30.1	9.6
1972	167.0	30.8	10.0
1973	178.9	31.8	11.3
1974	194.8	32.9	11.6
1975	195.3	33.5	12.3
1976	207.7	34.1	12.4
1977	204.2	34.4	12.6
Percent change 1965–1977	120.5%	30.3%	

Source: American Hospital Association, *Hospital Statistics, 1978.*

are complying with this mandate. While hospital inpatient admissions have increased at roughly a *2 percent* annual rate in this decade, hospital óutpatient clinic visits have risen at nearly a *7 percent* rate (see Table 6).

Except for 1966–1967, when the introduction of Medicare and Medicaid produced a short-lived decline in the share of hospital expenses going to outpatient services, in the past decade a growing share of additional patients seeking services is obtaining them on an outpatient basis. Since 1973, in fact, the cost of inpatient services has been rising at a 3–6 percent faster rate than the cost of providing an equivalent level of services on an outpatient basis. As outpatient clinics take on more of the lower-cost services for which hospitalization is optional, the average difficulty of inpatient cases—and the relative cost of inpatient services—will continue to climb over the next decade.

With the average difficulty of inpatient cases increasing, there has been a marked shift in the composition of hospital facilities over the past ten years. More and more general medical/surgical hospital beds are being converted to specialized units to accommodate the increasingly difficult cases. Ninety-one percent of the nation's 1.55 million hospital beds in 1971 were general medical/surgical beds. Fewer than 85 percent of the nation's beds are today general medical/surgical, due largely to a decrease in the number of general beds from 1.4 million to 1.12 million because of closures and conversions. Most of the growth in hospital beds since 1971—and the lion's share of new bed construction—has been for specialized units such as intensive care, rehabilitation and respiratory therapy departments, and the like. The total number of specialized beds has risen more than 70 percent in the last six years.

This shift in the service intensity of hospitals toward the more difficult cases has also been exacerbated by the general aging of the population. In the years ahead, as the baby-boom age group grows toward old age, an ever greater percentage of the population will be subject to the health problems of the elderly. From 1965 to 1975 the hospital utilization rate of the population as a whole rose only slightly, from 152 per 1,000 population to 164, an increase of less than 8 percent. The utilization rate of the population over sixty-five, however, has increased at a rate *better than seven times that of the total population.* Even in 1965 the aged hospital utilization rate, at 264 per 1,000, was 74 percent higher than the population as a whole. By 1975, however, this disparity was 125 percent; the admissions rate for persons sixty-five and over had jumped to 363 per 1,000 (see Table 7).

TABLE 7 **Hospital Admissions for the Aged and Nonaged 1965–1976**

Year	Aged Admissions	Nonaged Admissions	The Aged as Percentage of Total
1965	4,871,000	26,319,000	15.6%
1976	7,761,000	30,985,000	20.0%
Percent change:	59%	17.7%	

Source: Department of Health, Education, and Welfare, *Health, 1978.*

If anything, utilization rates viewed alone seriously *understate* the impact of the aged on the total hospital cost problem. Because of their heightened risk of serious disease and organ failure, the per capita cost for hospital care for the aged is nearly *three times* that for the population as a whole. Not only are they admitted more than twice as frequently as the population as a whole, but the average cost per admission, even with a 25 percent shorter average stay, is at least 25 percent higher than the national average for all age groups (Table 8).

The pressure which the aging of the population will continue to place on per-admission hospital costs is being felt even now. In both 1977 and 1978 the rate of admission of those below the

TABLE 8   Average Cost per Admission
of the Aged and Nonaged
1977

U.S. average	$1,561
Aged 1–64	1,463
Aged 65 and over	1,951

Source: Department of Health, Education, and Welfare, *Health, 1978.*

age of sixty-five grew rather slowly, at a rate of 1.6 percent per year. The rate of admission for those sixty-five and over, however, is accelerating—up 5.1 percent in 1977 and 5.9 percent in 1978.

The cost of increasing hospital admissions will continue to rise as a result of the increasing severity of the average hospital caseload and the overall aging of the population. With the likelihood increasing that the marginal patient will be seriously ill, the average hospital's revenue today will be inadequate to provide care for the patients of the 1980s.

The "Waste Substitution" Fallacy: Static Efficiency Losses and Dynamic Growth

The task confronting regulatory initiatives to cut hospital costs, in light of the evidence of pervasive continuing demands for increased intensity of hospital services, must perforce be to locate "waste" in hospital operations and then to cash that waste out in order to finance future demands on the system for increased hospital service capabilities. Yet while the perception of pervasive waste in our hospital system is nearly universal, it is impossible to expect hospitals to locate sufficient waste in their own institutions to finance every conceivable future demand on the system. It is true that not all hospitals are well managed and that the system is plagued to some extent by excessive investment in only facilities and equipment. Yet lowering utilization of existing facilities, the feasible regulatory approach to waste reduction, will have only a marginal effect on hospital operating costs while severely increasing unit costs for the remaining users.

Even those gains that *can* be achieved in reducing total system costs, moreover, will not be a very helpful means for hospitals to comply with revenue controls computed on a percentage increase basis. This is because such utilization reductions are essentially *one-time savings.*

Suppose that a hospital manages through reduced utilization of existing facilities to meet the total expenditure-increase limits. For example, by reducing CT scan usage, eliminating routine preadmissions tests, and closing off a few rooms on the second floor, a hospital manages to hold its cost increase in a given year to 9.7 percent—resulting in total expenditures of $1.097 million, up from $1 million the year before.

If the hospital wishes to meet the revenue growth goals established for the next year, its rate of increase *will not be measured against its level of expenditures during the period before elimination of the allegedly wasteful practices.* Rather it will start with the "lean and tight" total expenditure level it achieved in the prior year. In other words, *none* of the supposed efficiency gains will help the hospital achieve the limits in subsequent years. Unless more "waste" is located and eliminated, the hospital will be forced to constrain service increases in that year over and above the rate of inflation in its new lean budget.

The practical effect of using the "waste substitution" method to achieve compliance with revenue controls is that hospitals will be forced to preside over a shrinking service capability year after year. For hospitals that start out being relatively efficient, this will be particularly problematic. They will have less cutting to do to hold their rates of increase down, on average, but they will also have far fewer places where cuts can be safely made.

The perverse effect here is that in terms of potential for increased service intensity, wasteful institutions will be far better off than institutions that have carefully controlled their service capacity growth in the past. Hospitals with currently low occupancy rates will be offered considerable latitude to convert their empty general beds to more effective uses. On the other hand, hospitals that are now operating close to optimum efficiency will be hard-pressed to improve their services at all. If their individual price inflation experience significantly exceeds the rate of price increases indemnified by the allowable increase formula, efficient hospitals will be forced to *restrict* services to bring their operations within expense increase limits. This problem is endemic to the revenue cap approach. Because it concentrates on expense and charge rate changes from year to year rather than concentrating on the level of services actually being offered, the revenue cap is blind to efficiency or inefficiency. Because it is computed on a percentage basis, hospitals that are now spending the most will be allowed the largest increases. Hospitals with relatively modest expenditures will be allowed to increase the least. The inevitable response to the revenue cap for the proportion of hospitals that *are* relatively efficient is to constrain services offered and turn people away. This is amply demonstrated by the experience of hospitals in the great majority of states with mandatory control programs now underway (Stockman and Gramm 1979, p. 34).

THE IMPLICATIONS OF
MANDATORY REVENUE CONTROLS

The implicit purpose of revenue limit programs is to provide the federal government with leverage it can use to affect the management decisions of hospitals. Revenue caps alone do not provide sufficient control to ensure that hospitals will cut their costs by cutting waste. In fact, the revenue controls generally provide a counterincentive to eliminating unneeded hospitalizations and services. Admitting people who do not need a lot of services is an ideal money-maker for hospitals. Faced with absolute revenue limits, hospitals are unlikely to get rid of questionable technology. They *are* likely to do everything in their power to get rid of high-cost patients.

Certainly hospitals would never throw the most seriously ill into the streets to improve their balance sheets. The medical profession generally has strong ethical principles in this regard which ensure that hospitals will do the best they can to serve the nation's acute health care needs regardless of allowable revenues. Yet at the margin, in those circumstances where the hospital has latitude, there will be a continual bias toward providing services where expected revenues most exceed delivery costs.

The only way that the federal government could combat the incentive which its own regulatory program would create is to gain some degree of operating control over the institution. By using the considerable discretion that must be granted lest the program lose all appearances of fairness, the federal government can put the screws to those facilities that, in its august opinion, are responding improperly to the clarion call for health care expenditure reductions. Once forced by the revenue limits to plead for mercy, hospitals will be forced to accept the HEW Secretary's nonnegotiable demands for operational changes.

The main question, therefore, is whether establishing the secretary as a hospital czar is the most desirable or appropriate way to ensure that the American people receive the greatest value for the dollars they spend on hospital services.

While the health care market is admittedly imperfect due to the unrestrained demand for hospitalization generated by current federal policy, this is an argument for *changing* that federal policy rather than adding a new layer of secretarial controls. As we have seen, the hospital system is currently fraught with problems because the incentives in the system are biased toward maximizing expenditures. Attempting to cap the system without changing the fundamental incentives of patients and physicians ordering services will only ensure that the quality of the product declines. Blanket revenue caps, because they fail to deal with the underlying problem of excessive demand for services, cannot possibly deliver on the promise of a quality product for fewer dollars. Such regulation can only ensure that expenditures keep rising while the product deteriorates.

In rejecting the revenue cap approach, the Congress set the stage for the development of policy responses to the problem of rising health care costs that attack the underlying problem of cost-conscious demand. In so doing, it has fundamentally altered the future of federal health policy. We are firmly convinced, given the past decade's desultory experiments in regulatory control, that such a change can only be for the better.

7

CHARLES E. PHELPS

Public Sector Medicine: History and Analysis

Indirect and direct subsidies on supply and demand sides of the market. Criteria used to judge NHI. The effect of Medicare and Medicaid. The role of price controls. Subsidizing private health insurance. VA, DOD, and SLG hospitals. The increase in supply of physicians and surgeons and their geographical diffusion. The advantage of decentralized control.

THE MAGNITUDE OF PUBLIC INVOLVEMENT IN THE MEDICAL SECTOR

The public sector of the United States has had a long and growing relationship with the finance and delivery of medical care

for many decades, although public involvement in this country
still remains considerably less than in most other developed
countries. Public participation has taken three forms which may
be characterized in terms of the directness of involvement. First
is an indirect subsidy—the exemption of certain medical care
(and medical insurance) providers from U.S. taxes, which often
carries with it exemption from state and local sales and property
taxes. Multiple direct subsidies also arise—among them the Hill-
Burton hospital construction program, medical school assistance, and support for biomedical research. These subsidies are
directed to the "supply side" of the market.

Second are indirect and direct subsidies on the "demand
side." The indirect subsidy arises through the tax deductibility
of medical expenses for persons with itemized deductions and
of personally paid health insurance premiums, as well as exclusion of employer-paid insurance premiums from the tax base itself. Direct subsidies to consumption have historically been
focused on subpopulations viewed as of lower income or more
in need of care, ranging from Maternal and Child Health programs to the much more extensive Medicare and Medicaid programs enacted in 1965.

Third, various governmental levels have provided medical
care directly. This form includes local city or county hospitals
and clinics through state general, mental, and tuberculosis hospitals and up to the Veterans' Administration (VA) hospital
system and the medical care systems operated by the Department of Defense (DOD).

Expenditures are largest for demand subsidies. Direct medical
payments accounted for over $40 billion per year in 1977 (ex-
trapolated to $60 billion per year in 1980 at 15 percent annual
growth rates). Of this amount, over $21 billion in 1977 ($32
billion extrapolated for 1980) arises through the Medicare program (Title 18 of the Social Security Act), and another $18
billion in 1977 ($27 billion by 1980) through the Medicaid pro-
gram (Title 19 of the Social Security Act). Workman's Compensation programs added $2.6 billion in 1977 ($4 billion by 1980).

There were also three important sources of indirect subsidies to demand for medical care through the tax system. Most important, the federal tax law provides that employer payments for health insurance premiums should not be taxed as income, an almost unique exception in tax treatment of employer-paid benefits. It has been estimated recently that this cost the federal treasury $8 billion in 1978 (and $13 billion in 1980; see Phelps 1980). Further, direct allowance of deductions for health insurance premiums and for direct medical expenses by individuals account for something near $6 billion in 1980.[1]

Direct operation of medical care services in the United States is substantial. State and local hospitals are the largest single class of public providers, accounting for one out of every four hospitals in the country, 15 percent of all hospital beds, and over 20 percent of all hospital admissions (American Hospital Association 1979). Total expenditure in these hospitals in 1977 was about $8 billion. Despite the more widespread fame of larger county and city hospitals, the most common state or local government (SLG) hospital in the United States is small (average of 120 beds), located in a rural area, and probably constructed or renovated through assistance of Hill-Burton hospital construction funds.

Although only 8 percent of these SLG hospitals are medical-school affiliated, these affiliated hospitals (most of which are large, urban hospitals in excess of 400 beds) account for one-third of all SLG hospital beds. Including hospitals with internship and residency programs, the fraction of all SLG hospital beds involved in some fashion in medical education or teaching programs rises to 40 percent.

The largest single hospital system in the United States is that operated by the Veterans' Administration, accounting for over 5 percent of all U.S. hospital beds, with annual operating expenditures for hospitals and other VA facilities in excess of $4.3 billion in 1977 (extrapolated to $6.5 billion in 1980). About 60 percent of these hospitals are affiliated with medical schools in a direct or limited teaching arrangement.

Table 1 summarizes these major categories of public involvement in medical care. Taken together, public sector activities accounted for nearly $84 billion in 1977, amounting to 51 percent of all private health expenditures. This fraction has grown considerably in the past several decades. From 1950 through 1965 government expenses represented a stable amount near 25 percent of total health expenses. Since the passage of Medicare and Medicaid—and with other public programs—this fraction has increased steadily in the past fifteen years to its current level.

More traditional accounting methods show the government to be involved in some 43 percent of all health expenses. The major difference here is inclusion of the subsidies to health insurance and medical spending arising through the federal income tax system. But it is important to include these amounts in assessing the extent of government involvement in medical care. Recent categories of expense growing most rapidly are those involving direct government payment for health care (e.g., Medicare) and these categories of indirect expenditure.[2]

This accounting documents the magnitude of public activity in U.S. medicine more fully than previous estimates and it shows the programs in which expenditures are most heavily concentrated. It helps focus further attention on those sectors of activity which, by virtue of their size, should be subjected to more careful investigation.

CRITERIA FOR PUBLIC SECTOR ACTIVITY

Public sector expenditures for medical care have been increasing steadily in this country for decades, rising from 14 percent of all medical expenditure in 1929 to present levels just above 50 percent. Current public activity is normally justified by desires to increase access to medical care for those previously unable to obtain care, and because health care is viewed as a "right" of all citizens regardless of ability to pay. Given this increasing public

TABLE 1   Major Categories of Public Sector Expenditure
in Health Care (1975)

Demand subsidies	Expenditure (billions)	
Medicare	$21.6	
Medicaid and other welfare	17.6	
Worker's compensation	2.6	
Income tax deduction of medical care	4.0	
Income tax deduction of health insurance premiums (personal)	2.0	
Employer-paid premium tax exemption	8.5	
Total—demand side expenditures		$ 56.3
Supply operations		
General federal, state, and local hospitals and other medical services	$8.3	
Veterans Administration system	4.3	
Department of Defense system	3.4	
Public health programs	3.7	
Total—supply side expenditures		19.7
Other federal/state/local		7.6
Total		$ 83.6
Total health spending in the United States		$162.8
Government as percent of total		51.0%

Sources: Gibson and Fisher 1978; Phelps 1980.

involvement as well as the potential for further increases if national health insurance is enacted, it seems reasonable to ask if existing programs have achieved their promised objectives. In particular:

—Has public involvement increased access for the disadvantaged?

—Has it evened the geographic distribution of available services?

—Has it contributed to the increase in the relative price of medical care in this country in recent years?

—In a general efficiency sense, what are the social welfare gains and costs? Is the correct type and quantity of care being provided?

—Have particular publicly operated supply organizations (e.g., SLG and VA hospitals) been efficient in an organizational sense? Are they delivering care for the least possible cost in relation to alternatives?

In the debate on national health insurance (NHI), it will be useful to analyze several major public programs in terms of these criteria in answering the following questions:

—Are past programs justified, and are there indications (such as market failure) that would justify further public involvement?

—What is the appropriate role for existing public sector medical activities under national health insurance?

—What would be the likely outcomes of various additional levels of public involvement through NHI?

THE DEMAND SIDE OF THE MARKET

The Medicare Program for the Aged

The Social Security Amendments of 1965 (Title 18) provided for the first time in U.S. history a comprehensive health insurance program available to an entire group of the general population (those sixty-five and older) regardless of income or ability to pay for care. This program has since been extended to encompass the permanently disabled and those with chronic kidney disease. The elderly were widely viewed as particularly disadvantaged with regard to medical care because of (a) the strong association between age and illness, (b) the generally low incomes of the aged, and (c) the low level of wealth accumulation by many of the aged. This population group is not only the sickest of any, but also the least able to pay for care out of current income or asset depletion. The Social Security program in general provided a major income transfer to the generation which suffered through the Great Depression, but the program is intended to become self-financing for those currently entering the labor market.[3] Medicare has furthered that process by providing for the elderly at no-charge hospital insurance (Part A), leading to annual hospital expenditure of $465 per enrollee financed through the plan,[4] and general medical/surgical insurance (Part B) at a charge considerably less than its actuarial value.[5]

The program's effects on medical care use have been dramatic. Hospital admission rates for the elderly rose nearly 25 percent after the introduction of Medicare, and the rate of surgical procedures rose 40 percent (Andersen ct al. 1972). Average length of hospital stays also rose considerably—which increased by nearly 50 percent the number of hospital days per person over sixty-five (Newhouse 1976). Physician office visits did not follow the same pattern, however. First, because of the deductible ($50 originally, later increased to $60 per year), demand by the elderly did not expand as much as it would have in its absence. Just over half of the Part B–enrolled persons meet the $60 annual deductible, and little change in demand is expected for those persons not meeting it (Newhouse, Phelps, and Schwartz 1974). Further, with the 20 percent copayment required of persons on the Part B program, increases in market prices for physician services will deter utilization somewhat. A concurrent widespread adoption of major-medical insurance for the under-sixty-five population probably increased effective demands on physicians considerably during the period, thereby increasing prices.

Another possibility is that physicians and elderly patients together decided that the most desirable form of medical treatment for some diseases had switched when improved financing was brought about by Medicare. Although the patient was required to pay the first day's room and board fee for the hospital, coverage was essentially complete for hospital expenses thereafter so long as the length of stay was not over sixty days (see below). Thus, although the coverage for physician services also generally improved for the elderly, the relative cost of treatment in the hospital (relative to outpatient treatment) may have fallen, making the hospital particularly attractive as a place of treatment. A substitution of hospital care for ambulatory care therefore may account for part of the increased hospital utilization and decreased use of physician services after the program was instituted.

An important distinction must be made between *demand* and *utilization* of medical care. Demand is the number of persons *trying* to obtain such care (at a given price, income distribution, etc.), whereas *utilization* is the amount of care actually received. If more persons are attempting to obtain care at a given price than there are services to be provided, then utilization will be less than demand. Since Medicare, Medicaid, and private insurance expansion all increased the demand for physician services during the late 1960s, one likely explanation for the fall in physician utilization by the elderly is that while their effective demands increased, those of other population groups increased even more, so that utilization by the elderly did not alter substantially—and in fact fell slightly.[6]

Despite the considerable income transfer under Medicare, the elderly still face substantial medical expenses not met by the federal program. A major reason is the structure of the program itself: for hospital stays in excess of sixty days, the patient must pay $45 per day through the ninetieth day; a lifetime reserve of sixty days' coverage (beyond the annual ninety-day coverage limit) requires daily payments of $90. Beyond that, no coverage exists for hospitalization. For physician and other services, a $60 deductible and a 20 percent copayment are structured into Part B, with no limit on copayments. Medicare thus has poor coverage for high-loss (but presumably lower-probability) events.[7] The resultant out-of-pocket expenditures arising for the elderly constitute what are commonly described as "catastrophic" expenses for a large fraction of the enrolled population. Data from a 1970 health care survey[8] demonstrate that for families with heads over sixty-five years of age, nearly half had out-of-pocket expenses exceeding 5 percent of their total family income and one-eighth had expenses in excess of 15 percent. Table 2 shows these data in more detail. These figures are probably conservative estimates of the extent of "catastrophic" expenses in 1975, because the relative price of medical care has increased considerably in the intervening years and demand for medical care is price inelastic.[9] Out-of-pocket expenses were approximately 40 percent of total expenses for these families.

TABLE 2   "Catastrophic Expense" for Families with Heads over Aged 65—1970

Definition of Catastrophic Expense	Percent of Families	Average Out-of-Pocket Expense (1970)	Out-of-Pocket Percent of Total Expense
5% of income	45	$417	38
10% of income	22	$548	37
15% of income	13	$679	40

Source: 1970 Center for Health Administration Studies Health Care Survey

General increases in medical prices suggest that the average out-of-pocket expense figures would be at least 50 percent higher in 1975 than in 1970, and the out-of-pocket expense as a percent of total expense has probably also increased because Medicare fee limitations to physicians have not increased as fast as medical prices in general.[10]

By 1976 over 60 percent of the Medicare population was purchasing private insurance to fill gaps in their Medicare coverage (Congressional Budget Office 1979). The structure of these plans clearly indicates a desire to eliminate the hospital copayments, i.e., the catastrophic expense aspect of hospitalization in general, to supplement Medicare payments to physicians and other providers (since the Medicare fee is often substantially less than the doctor's charge), and to provide out-of-hospital prescription drug coverage and to extend nursing home coverage (Ellenbogen 1974).

The Medicaid Program for the Poor

The other major public program providing "insurance" against medical expenses is the Medicaid program for low-income persons. Unlike Medicare, which is uniform for all states in the United States, Medicaid is a state-administered program financed by federal/state matching funds. Eligibility criteria, services covered, and administration of the plans are established by state governments and vary substantially from state to state. The unevenness of eligibility for Medicaid programs across states and the uncertainty of eligibility even within a given jurisdiction have led to growing public uneasiness about Medicaid as an appropriate vehicle for providing medical-expense protection for the low-income population. Nearly every national health insurance proposal before the Congress in the past decade, including the most recent, includes plans to federalize coverage for this population group (U.S. Senate Committee on Finance 1979).

Nevertheless, several features of this program deserve mention. First, and perhaps least understood, is that Medicaid (coupled with Medicare) has provided a significant leveling of coverage for medical service across income groups, particularly for physician ambulatory services. Table 3 shows that while strong association exists between income and the existence of *private* insurance coverage for ambulatory care, the distribution is very even when one adds public programs. Second, this leveling of financial coverage has led to a similarly even distribution of physician services per capita across income groups *for adults*, as shown in Table 4. Children of low-income families still receive significantly fewer physician visits than is true for other income groups.

TABLE 3 Proportion of Families with Coverage for Doctor Office Visits—1970
Type of Insurance Coverage

Income (% of sample)	Group	Nongroup	Private (subtotal)	Medicare	Medicaid	Public (subtotal)	Total
Under $3000 (18.5%)	0.05	0.03	0.08	0.39	0.10	0.49	0.57
$3000–4999 (12.3%)	0.17	0.02	0.19	0.23	0.06	0.29	0.48
$5000–6999 (12.4%)	0.24	0.03	0.27	0.11	0.02	0.13	0.40
$7000–9999 (18.2%)	0.35	0.02	0.37	0.04	0.01	0.05	0.42
$10,000–14,999 (12.8%)	0.42	0.01	0.43	0.01	—	0.01	0.44
$15,000+ (16.9%)	0.41	0.03	0.44	0.03	—	0.03	0.47
All incomes (100%)	0.28	0.02	0.31	0.13	0.03	0.16	0.47

Source: Charles E. Phelps, "Effects of Insurance on Demand for Medical Care," in Equity in Health Services: Empirical Analyses in Social Policy, Ronald Andersen et. al., eds. (Cambridge, Mass.: Ballinger Publishing Co., 1975).

TABLE 4   Physician Visits per Person Before and After
Medicare and Medicaid

Income	1963–64	1966–67	1973
Under $3,000	4.3	4.6	6.0
$3,000 - $7,000	4.5	4.1	5.2
$7,000 - $10,000	4.7	4.3	4.8
$10,000 - $15,000	4.8	4.5	4.9
Over $15,000	5.8	4.8	5.1
Age			
Under 65	4.3	4.1	4.8
65+	6.7	6.0	6.5

Source: Derived from data in *Vital Statistics, Series 10, No. 97, Physician Visits, Volume and Interval Since Last Visit, United States, 1971*, Table B and Table 1.

Effects of Medicare and Medicaid on the Price of Medical Care

It is demonstrably clear that public insurance programs for the elderly, disabled, and poor have significantly shifted the demand for care for these population groups, and this increased access has been correctly viewed as at least partially successful in meeting program objectives. But there is a cost, one measure of which is the direct expenditures for the programs (see Table 1). Another is the effect of these programs on prices for medical care for the U.S. population as a whole. The supply of medical services, particularly personal services such as physician and dental care, cannot expand rapidly in the face of new demands.[11] An inevitable result is that the price of medical care (relative to the price for other goods and services in the country) must rise. One estimate is that these combined public programs increased the demand for medical care by 10 to 15 percent (Newhouse, Phelps, and Schwartz 1974). The rate of price increases in the medical care sector doubled at the same time as these programs were introduced, as can be seen in Table 5. The period 1971–1974 reflects the impact of general wage and price controls on the industry. A remarkable fact is indicated in the price behavior of prescription drugs. Since Medicare provides no coverage for out-of-hospital prescription drugs, and since the supply of drugs can expand rapidly to meet new demands, it is to be predicted that drug prices would not be significantly altered by implementation of a new insurance program of Medicare/Medicaid dimensions, but the effect on physician and hospital prices is unmistakable.

The acceleration of medical care prices resulted from an increase in total demand for medical care that was modest because of the limited population covered by the new insurance programs. However, universal insurance coverage for the entire U.S. population is estimated to lead to much larger increases in demand than those generated by Medicare and Medicaid. For programs providing full coverage (no deductibles or coinsurance), the shift in *demand* for hospital care could rise by 5 to 15 percent and the *demand* increase for physician services could exceed 75 percent (Newhouse, Phelps, and Schwartz 1974; Phelps 1975). Such demand shifts could almost certainly not be met by existing supplies, particularly in the physician sector, and strong upward pressure on the price of medical care would inevitably result. Some of this pressure would be absorbed by nonprice rationing devices such as increased waiting times to see physicians, extended queues in physician offices, alterations in patterns of physician practice, or refusal of physicians to see certain types of patients (Newhouse, Phelps, and Schwartz 1974), but it appears inconceivable that anything except even more rapid price increases than today's would be observed.

Increases in the price of a specific good or service (such as medical care) typically serve multiple purposes. Aside from rationing available supplies among those seeking the service or good, increased relative prices typically draw new resources into the market, so that price increases are moderated in the long run and supply expands to meet the new demand. In the medical sector more extensive insurance coverage removes price as a rationing device, and other mechanisms must arise to allocate

TABLE 5 Annual Rates of Price Increase—Before and After
Public Health Insurance

Period	General CPI (1)	All Medical Care (2)	Hospital Room Rate (3)	Physicians' Fees (4)	Dentists' Fees (5)	Prescription Drugs (6)
1960–1965	1.3	2.5	5.8	2.8	2.4	−2.5
1965–1971	4.2	6.2	13.6	6.6	5.5	−0.1
1971–1974[a]	6.8	5.4	7.3	5.1	4.9	0.5

Source: Department of Labor Consumer Price Index

[a]Wage and price controls in effect during these years.

available care among those seeking it. In the short run, however, higher prices will not likely draw new resources into the field. Hospitals, typically organized as not-for-profit (or governmental) firms, may not respond to price increases in the "typical" market fashion. The number of physicians cannot expand rapidly in any case because of the long training period required, unless the United States dramatically alters its stance towards immigration of foreign-trained physicians. Nor is it likely that the hours worked by each existing physician would increase in the face of a price increase—the negative effects of increased income on labor supply appear to offset any incentives to work longer hours arising from the pure fact of higher prices (Sloan 1974, 1975). Thus a dramatic price increase for medical care would primarily transfer wealth from the population in general towards suppliers of medical services.[12]

The role of price controls is important in this context. If the government turns to price controls as a method of alleviating price increases, they may succeed in reducing the nominal price of care (as apparently occurred during the 1971–1974 price controls), but other rationing devices must arise which force the true market-clearing "price" *above* the free-market level. This principle holds whenever the demand curve is downward sloping and the supply curve is upward sloping. Figure 1 illustrates the result of price controls: A smaller quantity is supplied with the controls than in their absence, and the true market-clearing price is that where the quantity demanded intersects the quantity supplied. *Price controls raise, not lower, true transactions prices, but the controls are often illusory because they convert part of the full price into forms not entering the price index* (such as waiting time to obtain service).

The gasoline service station lines during the Arab oil embargo of 1973–1974, and again in the spring of 1979, dramatically demonstrated how full prices diverge from nominal "list" prices in a price-controlled market. In both of these cases price controls administered by the Department of Energy and its predecessor agencies prevented gasoline prices from rising to clear the

144 CHARLES E. PHELPS

FIGURE 1

MARKET-CLEARING PRICE WITH BINDING CONTROLS

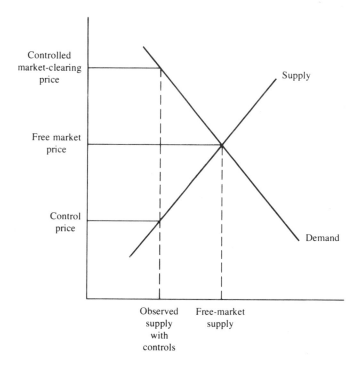

market, with the consequent lines exceeding three hours in length as the remainder of the "price" necessary to clear the market. As the rules allowed the pump price to rise, the lines were eliminated in both of these cases, and the market eventually cleared with only money prices rather than necessitating the considerable waste of time caused by the other circumstance.

Indirect Subsidies to Medical Insurance

One of the largest public interventions in the medical care sector has until recently been widely ignored—the subsidy to purchase of private health insurance in the federal tax structure. The subsidy was originally intended to provide incentives for families to purchase private health insurance, and this goal has been achieved for substantial segments of the population. The major subsidy arises because health insurance premiums paid by an employer do not enter the tax base for either personal or corporate income or payroll taxes. Like payroll taxes themselves, it has been generally established that most if not all of such premiums falls upon the worker—his wages are reduced to the extent that employer costs are increased by provision of such insurance. Therefore the appropriate tax rate to measure the subsidy is the marginal personal income tax of the worker (coupled with the payroll tax if the worker makes less than the payroll-tax maximum income). Two important consequences of such a subsidy are: (a) it is meaningless to those unemployed or with weak (part-time or intermittent) connections with the labor force and (b) it will rise with income because of the progressive nature of the personal income tax.

The effect of hinging a subsidy on labor-force participation is clearly seen in data in Table 6. Those without permanent labor-force ties are significantly less insured than those full-time employed.

That the subsidy increases substantially with income, and that this induces more purchase of insurance by recipients of that subsidy, is shown clearly in Table 7.[13] The fraction of families with employer group insurance rises from 80 percent for the lowest-income group to above 90 percent for upper-income groups. For those who actually have insurance, the per-family subsidy in 1975 increased from $48 per year to over $150 per year for upper-income groups. In 1980 the actual dollar figures will be more than double, i.e., ranging from $100 to $300 per family. The aggregate tax expenditure from this subsidy in 1980 will be near $12.5 billion (Phelps 1980).

A similar subsidy (though smaller in magnitude) arises from the deductibility of family-paid health insurance premiums and medical expenses from personal income for purposes of

TABLE 6 Private Health Insurance Enrollment Rates in 1970 for Families
(in percent)

Labor Force Status of Family	All Incomes	Poor (under $3000)	Near Poor ($3–5000)	Middle ($7–15,000)	High (above $15,000)
Full time	88	41	73	89	98
Part time	44	35	52	62	—
Unemployed	27	11	20	—	—
All persons in income class	76	38	65	82	95

Source: Charles E. Phelps, "The Distribution and Effectiveness of Private Health Insurance," testimony before U.S. House of Representatives Subcommittee on Public Health and Environment, *National Health Insurance—Implications*, (Washington, D.C.: U.S. Government Printing Office, 1974), Serial No. 93–69.

TABLE 7   Current Distribution of Employer-Paid Health Insurance Premiums by 1975 Income
and Average Subsidy per Family Unit

Income Class (1975 Income) of Tax Unit[a] ($)	(1) Families with Employer Group Insurance (%)	(2) Total Family Premiums per Insured Tax Unit[b] ($)	(3) Employer Premiums per Insured Tax Unit ($)	(4) Average Marginal Tax Rate, 1975 Tax Law (%)	(5) Subsidy per Insured Tax Unit ($)	(6) Aggregate Subsidy ($ billions)
0–3,000	8	336	219	22.69	48	0.018
3,000–5,000	26	329	204	28.95	60	0.085
5,000–7,000	53	356	214	31.49	68	0.214
7,000–10,000	66	441	266	31.73	84	0.614
10,000–15,000	81	641	433	31.36	137	1.863
15,000–20,000	88	619	406	30.63	124	1.095
20,000–50,000	92	629	436	34.06	151	1.581
>50,000[c]	100	720	720	50.3	362	0.047
All families	70	570	378	31.82	122	5.518

[a]Tax units are families and individuals, as defined for taxpaying purposes. See "New Tax Expenditures from Mandated National Health Insurance," Section IV, Mitchell and Phelps (1976).

[b]"Insured tax unit" means any family or individual with employer-group insurance. To obtain an estimate for all tax units in this income class, multiply the value shown in this column by the percentage given in col. (1).

[c]One observation.

Source: Mitchell and Phelps (1976)

calculating personal income tax liabilities. An analysis by Mitchell and Vogel (1975) shows that this subsidy leads to an additional tax expenditure of $2 billion for health insurance and about $1 billion for medical expenses *per se*. Extrapolation of these data to 1980 suggest an added tax expenditure of approximately $4 billion for health insurance and about $2 billion for medical expenses *per se*. Despite the requirement that out-of-pocket medical expenses must exceed 3 percent of family income before they become deductible, the progressive tax structure implies an *increasing* per-family subsidy to medical care from this mechanism. Like the elimination of employer-paid premiums from the tax base, the deductibility of family-paid premiums and medical expenses induces a subsidy positively correlated with family income.

The rationale for a continuing subsidy for the purchase of private health insurance is at best dubious if a universal health insurance plan is passed. The tax expenditures arising from the present subsidy are considerable and indeed are larger than the estimated new direct federal expenditures for some proposals before the Congress. Because the existing subsidy increases strongly with income, alteration of tax law to include employer-paid premiums in the tax base and removal of the deductibility of family-paid premiums and medical expenses is akin to implementing a new progressive tax which would provide an additional $18 billion (1980 dollars) in revenue annually for the U.S. Treasury.

THE SUPPLY SIDE—PUBLIC PROVISION
OF MEDICAL CARE

The Veterans Administration Medical System

The single largest organization in the United States providing medical care is the Veterans Administration (VA) hospital system. Composed of 120 general hospitals and 50 mental hospitals plus various clinics and rehabilitation centers, the VA is primarily devoted to providing treatment for military-related injuries and illnesses for U.S. military veterans. Treatment for other "unrelated" illnesses and injuries may be provided if facilities are available and if the veteran signs a statement that he cannot pay for care at alternative sources.

A separate medical system for veterans is desirable if specialized care for military injuries is not available in the private sector or if it can be provided with scale economies through the public sector. VA hospitals are also heavily involved in educating new physicians and in medical research. Thus if a particularly special role exists for the VA system in those capacities, there may be further justification for public production of care for veterans. As with any publicly provided program, however, one must also question whether the goals of the system (i.e., to assist veterans, particularly those with military-related injuries or illnesses) could be met more efficiently by other benefits—that is, if the optimal mix of benefits is being given. It is also appropriate to ask whether the public provider of the service is behaving efficiently, operating with the least possible cost to produce the benefit package chosen.

Two recent studies of the VA system have both raised serious questions about its continuing value. Both studies focus on three basic problems: First, providing benefits to veterans by requiring them to seek care in particular institutions is less valuable to veterans than allowing them free choice of source of care. Some veterans would prefer the cash equivalent to the care, because they can allocate cash to their own benefit more accurately than can the VA system. The VA system thus may be inefficient by providing the wrong benefit package.

Second, access to the care provided is very uneven across the veteran population. Because veterans often reside far away from any of the highly limited number of VA hospitals, the travel and time costs have made the VA more expensive to many veterans than private purchase of care from a local provider.

Third, the care may be provided in a technically inefficient manner; the VA system may be less efficient than the private hospital sector.

The concept of inequitable access arises almost necessarily in a general hospital system of 120 units spread about in a country which has 7,000 community hospitals in the same space. In rural or low-density areas prospective patients may have to travel hundreds of miles to reach a VA hospital. In fact, over 85 percent of all hospitalizations of veterans take place outside of the VA system.

Since the VA system does not charge any fee to veterans, bed space must be allocated by other mechanisms. The VA system relies heavily upon travel distance (as noted previously) and queuing to ration available services. Unfortunately, this type of rationing often makes it difficult for the VA to meet its first stated objective of providing care for military-related injuries and illnesses. Studies show 85 percent of the patients actually in the VA system are hospitalized for reasons not associated with military illness or injury. If a VA hospital is filled when a veteran with a military-connected medical problem presents himself, he must be turned away until a later date. The extent of this problem is not shown in available data.

The question of inefficiency is often posed regarding the VA system. On the one hand, there is a presumption of efficiency from the scale of operation on grounds that central purchasing of supplies, commonality of administration, uniform hiring policies, and other activities can lead to cost savings. Offsetting this, however, are the complexity of management, particularly of communications, and flexibility in dealing with specific problems, which tend to offset other scale economies. The question can only be resolved empirically, and that turns out to be a very difficult problem.

Making straightforward cost comparisons between VA hospitals and other community hospitals can run aground on several reefs. Most obvious is that the patient mix is considerably different. Most VA patients are hospitalized for illnesses of aging, poverty, or both. Many patients are admitted for psychiatric problems, including alcoholism and drug addiction. To be successful, a straightforward cost comparison between VA hospitals and other community hospitals must adjust for patient mix. The second problem in such a comparison is the allocation of joint costs. Since the VA system heavily engages in teaching (100 of the VA hospitals have a medical-school affiliation and most have some postgraduate training programs) as well as medical research, one must carefully assess joint cost effects when making efficiency comparisons. To my knowledge, no available data would allow a truly correct comparison to be made because the VA system does not keep accounting records conducive to joint cost studies. Several attempts have been made to assess average costs within the VA and other hospitals (Lindsay 1975; Starr 1973), but these inevitably result in average cost comparisons which arbitrarily allocate joint and fixed costs. The result makes the comparisons somewhat meaningless in a pure economic context.

Despite the difficulties in making appropriate cost comparisons, several indicators provide some evidence that the VA system is operating inefficiently. Foremost among these is the strong prohibition against ambulatory treatment built into the VA programs. Until recently, no patient with nonservice-connected illnesses could receive any ambulatory treatment through the VA program (recall that this group is 85 percent of total admissions). Recent modifications in the law have allowed the VA to provide ambulatory care for these patients before and after hospitalization, but treatment still requires hospitalization. Estimates reported by Lindsay (1975) and Starr (1973) are that between 10 and 20 percent of the patients in the VA system have no medical requirement for hospitalization.

The other major evidence on technical inefficiency is made on disease-specific costs of treatment. Table 8 shows the first measure of this, wherein age-specific lengths of stay for patients with specific diseases are compared from the VA system and

TABLE 8   Average Lengths of Stay in VA and Voluntary
Hospitals, by Surgical Procedure, for Patients
Age 50–64 except where Noted
(reported by days)

Procedure	VA	Voluntary	Ratio VA/ Voluntary
Pilonidal cyst (age 35–49)	15.7	5.8	2.7
Diabetes mellitus	19.0	9.0	2.1
Acute coronary occlusion	31.5	21.7	1.5
Hemorrhoidectomy	15.8	7.1	2.3
Tonsils and adenoids (age 35–49)	6.4	2.4	2.7
Duodenum ulcer	15.2	6.7	2.3
Appendicitis	12.1	6.9	1.8
Inguinal hernia	17.1	7.2	2.4
Gastroenteritis and colitis	11.1	7.7	1.4
Gallstones	26.5	11.9	2.2
Pyelitis, cystitis, nephritis	11.6	6.0	1.9
Kidney stones	18.6	8.2	2.3
Prostate	22.1	9.7	2.3

Source: Interagency Length of Stay Study Group (unpublished). Some results published in U.S. House of Representatives, Committee on Veterans Affairs, *Veterans Administration Hospital Funding and Personnel Needs,* 91st Congress, 2d Session, 1970, p. 3347. Reprinted in Lindsay (1975), p. 47.

community hospitals. For almost every disease listed, the length of stay in the VA hospital system is double that of the comparison community hospitals.

An accurate accounting of the costs of treating veterans would assess to the costs of each cure the time costs of the patient. Even if VA patient time is only valued at the minimum wage of $3.10 per hour, and then only for eight hours per day, this exercise suggests that true marginal cost should be raised by at least $24.80 per day (for both community and VA hospitals) when making cost comparisons. If a correct cost comparison were made using data from the VA system and from community hospitals, such a comparison would still overly favor the VA system by ignoring the costs of extended lengths of stay of patients. Adding patient costs (time costs) to the comparison will increase the likelihood that the VA system is inefficient.

Whither the VA?

After assessing the status of the VA hospital system carefully, taking into account the inequities arising from limited geographic dispersion of the VA system and from rationing by queues, the inefficiency in providing in-kind rather than more flexible benefits to veterans, and possible operational inefficiencies, both Starr (1973) and Lindsay (1975) have recommended a uniform health insurance plan for veterans rather than indefinite continuation of the VA system.

The role of the VA system under a national health insurance plan is not completely obvious. An important issue to be resolved is the true comparison of marginal costs of treating patients in the VA system. If, as present evidence suggests, VA hospitals use more of society's scarce resources to deliver a set bundle of services, then it seems illogical—with national health insurance providing uniform access for veterans to all hospitals—to continue to waste extra resources. This does not answer the question about specific treatment of military-related injuries or illnesses. The founders of the VA system assumed that a specialized hospital system could provide better care than community hospitals could.

The impact of national health insurance on even this function of the VA could be considerable. Since 85 percent of VA patients are not service-connected, and since the bulk of those are in the VA because of medical indigency, national health insurance could therefore remove a major element of the demand for VA services by existing patients. Evidence in Starr (1973) strongly suggests that veteran-patients prefer to be treated in community hospitals near their homes, even if they bear the cost, rather than go to the VA. Those who seek VA care primarily do so for financial reasons that would vanish under national health insurance. Could the VA system survive in such a circumstance even for treatment of service-connected disabilities alone? If demand for care in VA hospitals evaporated under national health insurance, as seems plausible, the answer is almost certainly "no." Congressional funding would undoubtedly evaporate with the demand and there would be strong pressure to change the purpose—possibly even the ownership—of the VA hospital facilities.

Four possibilities arise for the VA hospitals in this scenario. The first is that the hospitals close down. This is not only implausible for bureaucratic reasons, but a marked waste of a useful resource. The second and most plausible outcome is that the VA alter its style of medical care, reducing patient length of stay, offering better combinations of ambulatory care and inpatient care, and higher quality medical care. This would require substantial changes in VA staffing, a serious problem with present operation of the system (see Starr 1973), and probably a major modification of payments to physicians. The third possibility is that the VA hospital system expand service from veterans to the entire population. In other words, the VA could become a federally operated general, psychiatric, or geriatric hospital system. The fourth option is that the VA could transfer ownership of the VA hospitals to local communities or to private organizations for operation as community hospitals.

The choice between these last two alternatives rests on operational efficiency grounds—whether scale economies of operation of a large system of hospitals offsets inherent management, communication, and flexibility problems. If smaller systems are desirable, then a federally operated community-hospital chain is probably not the appropriate choice. Whatever the choice, it appears that any systematic planning for national health insurance should logically include decisions about the role or disposition of the VA hospital system. It seems unlikely that continuing operation of the VA system in its present role will be the best use of those resources if a national health insurance plan brings universal coverage to the veteran population.

Finally, regarding the VA role in medical education, it is obvious that for any role of the current VA hospitals aside from direct closure there is no particular reason why the teaching operations of the VA could not be continued or even enhanced.

Indeed, one could make the argument that medical education would be more appropriate in a facility which treated a broader segment of the population (for example, one including females) than the current VA system includes. Thus alternative roles for the VA under national health insurance may be even more beneficial to society from the viewpoint of medical education.

Department of Defense Hospitals

Aside from the VA, the other major federal provider of medical care is the health care system of the various branches of the Department of Defense (DOD). Each of the major military services (army, navy, air force) operates extensive hospital and ambulatory care centers at military bases throughout the world, with a heavy concentration in the United States. Their primary purpose is to provide care for active-duty personnel. An obvious requirement also exists for standby capacity in case of wartime increases in demands on the systems. A secondary role is to provide care on a space-available basis for dependents of active-duty personnel, and then for retired personnel and their dependents.

Operating in parallel with the DOD medical systems is a separate health insurance program, the Civilian Health and Medical Program of the Uniformed Services (CHAMPUS), which provides coverage similar to a typical major-medical policy for dependents and retired personnel.[14] With this coverage dependents and retired personnel can seek care in the private medical sector in the United States, although it has recently been required that patients be cared for at a military facility if one within forty miles of the person's residence has available space and manpower. Particularly because of the overlapping DOD medical systems and private care availability through CHAMPUS, one would expect the DOD systems to behave at least as a partly competitive hospital system rather than as an independent system unaffected by any potential competition.

The DOD medical systems present a unique contrast to the VA in terms of operating problems, impacts of national health insurance upon the system, and lessons to be learned from current operations.[15] Regarding current operations, the most common criticisms of the DOD systems are (1) excess capacity, particularly in terms of inpatient beds, and (2) unnecessary duplication of facilities arising because there is no single unified system but rather three separate ones. The problem of excess capacity is easy to document, but it may be an inherent feature of a military medical system and therefore not of concern. Many of the DOD hospitals were constructed during World War II and the Korean War, and capacity was intentionally established at a level to care for wounded servicemen in an extensive war. Much of this *constructed* capacity will of course be redundant in times of peace, because demands on the system are much lower. Congressional hearings dramatically pointed out that the DOD hospitals were operating at less than 45 percent of constructed capacity (U.S. House of Representatives 1974), with slight variation across the three armed services. However, occupancy rates of *operating* beds were near those observed in regular community hospitals, as shown in Table 9. Occupancy rates fell as the Vietnam War ended, but they returned to prewar levels by 1974 when the number of operating beds declined to half the peak levels of 1969. Average occupancy in nonprofit community hospitals in this same period ranged from 77 to 81 percent. Even this comparison is slightly misleading, however, because of the inherently low occupancy rates for smaller hospitals; many of the DOD hospitals, particularly those of the air force, are small by nature because of the lower numbers of personnel at particular military bases.

The question of duplication across armed services is a two-edged sword. The obvious charge is that such duplication increases costs of operation which could be eliminated by moving towards a tri-service unified system. A recent congressional investigation of the DOD medical systems related multiple incidents in which apparently unnecessary cross-hauling of patients

TABLE 9 Department of Defense Hospital Occupancy Levels

Fiscal Year	Operating Beds	Occupied Beds	Occupancy Rate of Operating Beds (percent)
1969	57,477	43,610	76
1970	54,899	38,491	70
1971	48,846	32,438	66
1972	40,178	26,969	67
1973	36,048	24,210	67
1974	30,989	23,818	77

Source: U.S. House of Representatives (1974), p. 7.

had arisen because of the parallel systems operated by the three services. The other side of this story, however, relates to the inherent flexibility of smaller organizations, which suggests that offsetting savings may arise from more compact lines of authority, from the ability to undertake special procedures to deal with particular problems, etc. No data exist to assess accurately which effect dominates the military medical systems.

Another important characteristic of bureaucratic agencies involves incentives for innovation. Niskanen (1968) has argued that competition among bureaucracies should lead to desirable innovation of technology and cost-saving methods that are difficult for a single, larger bureau. Certain characteristics of the DOD hospitals, particularly when contrasted with the VA system, suggest this has occurred.

A major problem now facing the DOD medical systems is the diminishing availability of physicians. When the military draft was abandoned, physician manpower in the military continued at previous levels for several years because of prior service commitments of many physicians, both those in the services and those with service commitments through the "Berry Plan."[16] These physicians are not now available in large numbers, and physician supply to the DOD systems has fallen off markedly. Patient load has not diminished proportionately because the DOD medical systems care not only for active-duty personnel and their dependents but for significant numbers of retirees and their dependents. Faced with this approaching "crunch," the DOD medical systems, particularly that of the air force, have actively moved towards alternative delivery modes, especially for ambulatory care. The air force medical system, for example, actively uses paramedical personnel with two years of specialized training as direct substitutes for general practitioners in many medical clinics, with apparently very good success and patient acceptance.

One reason why the DOD systems have been able to innovate in this way is that they are relatively unbound by state and local prohibitions on alternative forms of medical practice. Many states directly prohibit, and every state heavily regulates, the conduct of medical care by persons other than licensed physicians, and the private sector has exhibited a marked reticence to engage the services of physician assistants (PAs) and other paramedical personnel (Reinhardt 1972). The contrast between the smaller, quasi-competitive DOD medical systems and the more unified VA system is quite striking. While no formal studies of the efficacy of the PAs are yet available, preliminary indications are that the air force and other service experiments will be successful in reducing costs and maintaining patient satisfaction; but the experiment is still in progress. Although each PA nominally operates under the direct supervision of a licensed physician and the PAs are taught and strongly encouraged to request physician consultation on difficult cases (or to refer the patient to a physician directly), the full results of the program—particularly its impact on patients' health—have not yet been assessed. One important lesson from the DOD medical systems may eventually be that restrictive state laws prohibiting or restricting PA activity are a costly and largely ineffective way to control quality.

The role of the DOD medical systems under national health insurance is more straightforward to understand than is that of the VA. Because current CHAMPUS health insurance for dependents and retirees is now quite generous (more so than many proposed NHI plans, in fact), none of these plans would likely alter the demands upon the DOD medical systems significantly. Active-duty personnel account for roughly a quarter of all inpatient and ambulatory visits in the DOD systems; more than another third come from their dependents, with the remaining visits coming from retired personnel and their dependents. Dependents and retirees are now required to seek care in a DOD hospital or clinic if they reside within forty miles of such a facility before they can use their CHAMPUS benefits (a procedure designed to increase utilization of the "excess capacity" of the hospital system). If national health insurance were implemented, however, it is unlikely that many of these people would find their insurance coverage increased beyond that of CHAMPUS, so there would be no incentives for them to change their sources of care from those currently sought. Indeed, if national health insurance raised demand in the private sector substantially, thereby increasing the queues and other nonprice rationing mechanisms in that sector, more patients—not fewer—would seek care in the DOD system and the patient load might increase slightly. Thus there is little reason to expect a national insurance plan will alter the behavior or incentives facing the DOD system, and it would probably continue operation in substantially the same manner with or without a national plan.

State and Local Government Hospitals

State and local government (SLG) hospitals form an important portion of the total hospital supply in the United States and account for roughly one-fifth of all short-term hospital admissions and more than one-quarter of all hospital outpatient visits. The market share of SLG hospitals has remained remarkably stable over time in recent decades, despite the considerable impact of Medicare and Medicaid on the abilities of low-income and elderly persons to purchase care at alternative sources. As shown in Table 10, the market share of SLG hospitals for inpatient

TABLE 10   Market Shares for Hospital Admissions
             and Outpatient Visits (in percent)

Year	Not-for-profit		For-profit		State and Local Government	
	Admissions	OPV	Admissions	OPV	Admissions	OPV
1960	73	—	7	—	20	—
1965	72	65	7	4	21	31
1970	72	68	7	4	21	28
1978	71	68	8	4	21	28

Source: Derived from American Hospital Association (1979), Table 1.

care has actually increased slightly since these social insurance programs were introduced in 1965, although their share of ambulatory (outpatient department and emergency room) visits fell from a peak of 33 percent of the market in 1964 (not shown in Table 10) to the 28 percent level in 1978. It was widely believed that the passage of Titles 18 and 19 of the Social Security Act would draw the old and the poor out of SLG hospitals and into the "mainstream" of American medicine—the not-for-profit community hospital. Clearly this has not happened, and an important lesson is to be drawn from this experience for future consideration of national health insurance.

To understand why SLG hospitals have remained competitive at least in the inpatient sector, it is useful to remember the basic role of these hospitals in the U.S. medical care sector. The market share of SLG hospitals in inpatient admissions has been stable at 20 percent at least since World War II. These hospitals have been the "health insurance policy of last resort" for many low-income and elderly U.S. citizens (often overlapping groups), providing care at little or no charge for those persons who were without private health insurance and/or could not afford private hospital treatment.

SLG hospitals have also been a keystone in U.S. medical education, with nearly 40 percent of the SLG hospital beds in the country involved directly in medical education. The large, medical-school-affiliated, county hospital was an important training site for many of the physicians and nurses now in practice in the United States. It was commonly understood that patients arriving for free care in these institutions would be available as "teaching patients" for physicians in training. It was the usual practice, for example, that surgery in these hospitals would be undertaken by residents and interns with the assistance of medical students rather than the usual practice in private teaching hospitals of having surgery performed by the attending staff with the assistance of interns and residents. The belief was widely held after the passage of Medicare and Medicaid that the patients in these institutions would seek care in the private hospitals in their communities because they would probably be (a) closer, (b) nicer facilities, and (c) providers of better medical care (or at least more direct care by physicians who had completed their training).

Data in Table 10 make clear that the anticipated mass exodus did not occur. One reason for this, of course, was that although Medicare and Medicaid did indeed provide a substantial increase in coverage for the target populations, significant financial liability remained for some patients (see Table 2), particularly those with extended lengths of hospital stay. Thus some inherent demand probably remained for "the insurance policy of last resort," even with these social programs.

It also appears from available data that SLG hospitals responded to the challenge with substantial upgrading of the medical care provided. The most dramatic indicator is the behavior of staffing patterns, as shown in Table 11. Before Medicare and Medicaid improved the financial health of SLG hospitals their staffing patterns were about 93 percent of the standard set by not-for-profit hospitals. Yet by 1977 SLG hospitals were employing 5 percent *more* employees per patient day than were not-for-profit hospitals, and this despite a massive increase in

TABLE 11   Staffing Patterns in Private and Public Hospitals

Year	Not-for-Profit Hospitals (1)	State and Local Government Hospitals (2)	Ratio (2)/(1)
1960	2.31	2.15	.93
1965	2.52	2.34	.93
1970	2.92	2.98	1.02
1977	3.69	3.87	1.05
1977 staff levels / 1965 staff levels	1.46	1.65	

employees per patient in the not-for-profit sector. Put differently, while not-for-profit hospitals increased their number of employees *per patient* by 46 percent between 1965 and 1977, SLG hospitals had a commensurate increase of 65 percent.

Another factor is locational. In many low income and rural communities SLG hospitals are the only sources of care, and the mere travel distance to alternative sources of care may make it unlikely that the prospective patient would change sources of care, even with better insurance available.

The budgets of SLG hospitals underwent a dramatic transformation with the advent of Medicare and Medicaid. Previously these hospitals operated almost entirely on funds allocated directly from local governmental authorities, with few if any direct patient revenues. Today these hospitals directly bill the Medicare and Medicaid programs for hospital services rendered, thus providing a significant portion of operating costs. Physician staffs of these hospitals have frequently formed group practices exclusively for the purpose of billing Part B of Medicare and Medicaid as well, providing still further funds for hospital operation.

These new revenues have served to make SLG hospitals more independent from local fiscal authorities and, because the hospitals depend upon maintaining their patient satisfaction to a considerable extent to maintain revenues, made the hospitals more responsive in their operations. Many SLG hospitals thus now compete directly with private sector hospitals rather than, as previously, serving as a last-resort medical care source for those who could not pay private hospital costs.

If this conjecture is true, it raises the obvious question of whether it is desirable for the public sector to be involved in providing a service. Public provision of services in areas such as defense, police and fire protection, education, and possibly in water supply are justified because of "externalities"—situations in which every person has an incentive to underproduce (or underdemand) the product, or because production is characterized by increasing returns to scale over the relevant range.[17] The legitimacy of either reason for medical care is unclear. If society feels an obligation to provide (at least a minimum amount of) medical care to all citizens—an obligation often expressed by declaring that "health care is a right"—it still does not follow that public provision is necessarily good. If universal insurance comes into being, and particularly if such insurance includes extensive benefits, the case for public provision becomes weaker and weaker.

The crucial question is whether any economic justification exists for providing governmental subsidies to continue the operation of specific institutions providing medical care. Once the public becomes satisfied that national health insurance meets the social goal of "equitable access to medical care," it would appear that questions of efficiency should dominate the decision about what types of organizations should provide the care. If governmental hospitals required continuing subsidies to operate in such an environment, that would constitute clear evidence of inefficiency, unless it could be demonstrated that there were some particular economies of scale in hospital operations that led to private underproduction. While the evidence is scanty and often based upon analyses of average (rather than marginal) costs of output, there appear to be eventual diseconomies of scale in hospital operation (Berki 1972). There is therefore a presumption that no governmental intervention is required to offset any problem of long-run declining marginal costs.

It is likely that if a universal health insurance plan is passed, SLG hospitals will continue to adapt just as they did in the new environment presented by Medicare and Medicaid. The local control and noncentralized management (relative, say, to the VA or DOD systems) in all likelihood promote such adaptability. The resolution of continued government subsidy to such operations, just as in the case of the VA medical system, will be an important issue if and when universal health insurance is passed. For continued public subsidies for medical care by state and local governments to be efficient economically, a clear case must be established that private hospitals and clinics are not providing the right amounts and kinds of care. Otherwise, more resources will be used to deliver U.S. medical care than are required and public supply will reduce overall welfare. This case has not yet been made.

PUBLIC INTERVENTION IN PHYSICIAN SUPPLY

Another form of government intervention in U.S. medicine, while not included in the discussion or the tables above, deserves mention. Over the past decade the output of U.S. medical schools has nearly doubled, primarily as a result of manpower program efforts through capitation and subsidy to the medical schools. The effects of this massive increase in physician manpower are just now being documented (Schwartz, Newhouse, Bennett, and Williams 1979; Newhouse 1979). The consequences of this increase in physician supply are much as one might predict from a normal working market, despite a considerable literature in health economics to the contrary.

The added manpower has resulted primarily in an outward diffusion of physicians from larger cities into smaller and smaller cities and rural areas as market pressures force the new physicians to seek business in previously unserved areas. This has occurred in virtually every specialty as well as in "family-practice" oriented specialties. The diffusion of physicians into more rural areas has extended to a degree that virtually all towns of over 30,000 population are represented by each of the five major specialties—internal medicine, surgery, radiology, pediatrics, and obstetrics/gynecology—whereas in 1960 only 58 percent of such towns were equally covered by board-certified specialists. Table 12 portrays the patterns of diffusion for the past seventeen years.

TABLE 12   Diffusion of Board-Certified Specialists since 1960: Percent of Communities in Which All Five of the Largest Board-Certified Specialties[a] Are Represented

	Population Range in Thousands						
Year	2.5-5	5-10	10-20	20-30	30-50	50-200	200+
1960	0	1	3	30	58	85	100
1970	0	1	11	44	80	92	100
1977	0	4	18	71	95	95	100

Source: Schwartz, Newhouse, Bennett, and Williams 1979.
[a]Internal medicine, surgery, radiology, pediatrics, obstetrics/gynecology.

CONCLUDING REMARKS

Public intervention in medicine has risen steadily over time, and by the mid-1970s had surpassed 50 percent of total health care expenditures in this country when properly calculated. The major portion of this intervention has been directed towards increasing the demand for medical services by specific population groups, notably the poor and the elderly. Simultaneously, a long history of public supply of medical care has primarily focused either on these same groups or on former members of the armed forces in compensation for their services. National health insurance would extend the public role in the health sector even further and, at least for most proposals before the Congress, would further specialize the public involvement into stimulation of demand for care. Under these circumstances, long-run expansion of the medical care sector will be required to keep per-unit prices from rising. While public control on total dollar expenditure could be used to keep "lids" on total resource use, it would then be true that other resources—such as patient time— would be required to ration available care.

Under any circumstances, the economic efficiency of the actual production of medical care may be significantly affected by how much production is undertaken in public hospitals. One possible lesson to be learned from existing public production of hospital care is that decentralized control of such agencies appears to allow more flexibility in response to new environments than is possible in centralized bureaus.

8

JACK A. MEYER

Proposals under Consideration*

What lies behind the promotion of national health insurance. Costs and benefits included in suggested programs. Comprehensive or catastrophic coverage? The Carter plan. Bills and proposals by Senators Kennedy, Long, Dole, Danforth, Domenici, Durenberger, Schweiker, and Representative Ullman. Financial problems, private and public. An evaluation.

All major proposals for national health insurance (NHI) provide minimum standard benefits both for those now uninsured and for those whose coverage would be altered. The major

*The author would like to thank Eileen M. Barbera for valuable research assistance.

differences in benefits partly concern the extent of the standard package—some bills limiting it to catastrophic coverage and others extending it to more routine services. Another issue concerns whether the package should be mandated or encouraged through incentives.

In addition to differences in benefits, proposals differ in their approaches toward drawing additional resources from other uses to meet increases in demand associated with NHI. In the current climate of budget austerity, such differences are sometimes portrayed as alternative ways to increase health care coverage without significantly increasing the budget deficit. But if improved care for some people is to be achieved without cutting back care for others, spending for health care must increase, and this is true regardless of whether the costs appear as rising charges and incomes for providers or as increased inconvenience and waiting time for services.[1]

Faced with a conflict of values—on the one hand wanting to provide more insurance while, on the other, wanting to moderate costs of health care—proponents accompany their NHI proposals with recommended structural changes in the health care system, changes designed to offset or contain the increased spending resulting from broader insurance coverage. Despite similarities in benefits, NHI proposals differ sharply in their basic strategies for keeping a lid on spending.

Two fundamentally different approaches to cost containment distinguish one group of proposals from another. One emphasizes the need to control providers—doctors and hospitals. It features controls on physician fees, limitations on hospital revenues, and restrictions on hospital capital expenditures. The other strategy is keyed on changes in the tax incentives related to the purchase of insurance and on the need for increasing competition among different types of insurance arrangements and delivery mechanisms. Advocates of such reforms argue that they will reduce the "waste" component of demand and thus allow for increased demand by the underserved without significantly increased spending.

The first approach diagnoses the problem in terms of excess capacity (e.g., unneeded hospital beds) alleged to be caused by the power of providers to increase supply even if demand is lacking; its sponsors believe that controls on providers, as excess capacity is utilized, will allow demand to increase without raising costs. The second approach suggests that, through incentives to economize on resources rather than to waste them, we can accommodate an increased demand for some by cutbacks in spending across the general population.

These different approaches—one geared to controls on the supply side, one geared to incentives on the demand side—reflect a basic division of opinion among health care economists regarding the nature of the market for medical care. Those favoring more regulation of providers stress the importance of inherent "market failure" in medical markets and believe that supply creates its own demand; the answer, then, is to control supply. Those who favor tax reform and incentives for consumers to shop for health insurance stress the importance of "regulatory failure" in health care markets and argue that the alleged excess spending for health could be corrected through altering the system of signals and incentives to which providers, patients, and insurers respond.

The first group emphasizes the unique nature of the health care market. It suggests that consumers' ignorance leads them to rely on doctors for decisions about treatment, rendering the conventional economic theory of consumer demand relatively useless in assessing the problem of health care costs. According to this view, notions of consumer sovereignty make little sense in a world where the patient, in effect, abdicates decision-making to various physicians who act as agents. These physicians are believed to "control" demand and, in the view of most advocates of this position, strive to achieve a "target income" either through fee setting or through influencing the number of tests and office visits, the length of stays in hospitals, and so on.

The second school of thought believes that the forces of competition—if not impeded by institutional constraints—can work in medical markets, albeit in a different manner from those in most other markets. Proponents of this view argue that health care consumers frequently have enough information to generate outcomes as close to competitive equilibrium as would occur with most other services. The fact that patients obviously have little or no influence over *emergency treatment* does not mean that they are without influence in the case of relatively routine care or that incentives to economize on the purchase of health *insurance* will be ineffective.

DIFFERENCES IN BENEFITS

The preceding conceptual schemes are translated into an array of proposed national health insurance programs. First, the proposals of President Carter and Senator Edward M. Kennedy would *mandate* a *comprehensive* health care plan for all Americans. The basic difference in these proposals is not in the type of services that would be covered by insurance, but in the timing or "phasing in" of the coverage. Second, proposals by Senators Long (S. 760) and Dole, Danforth, and Domenici (S. 748) would *mandate* coverage for *catastrophic* expenses associated with major illnesses, but other elements of insurance coverage would remain discretionary. Third, Senators Durenberger and Schweiker and Representative Ullman would provide tax incentives *encouraging but not mandating* the provision of catastrophic insurance. All of these bills, of course, are subject to substantial revision as the legislative process unfolds.

President Carter's National Health Plan

The Carter administration's national health plan (NHP) would eventually provide health insurance coverage for all Americans.[2] In the initial phase of a five-stage plan, the program would provide unlimited hospital and physician services for the poor who are covered by Medicaid. It would also provide fully subsidized health benefits to an estimated 10.6 million people not covered by Medicaid but whose income is less than 55 percent of the federal government's poverty standard, and to another 4.0 million whose health expenses cause them to "spend down" to this 55 percent line. For an estimated 24.0 million nonpoor aged and disabled people—the present Medicare recipients—cost-sharing would be limited by an annual cap of $1,250 per person, the current limit on fully subsidized hospital days would be removed, and all physicians would be mandated to accept assignment from the government with no extra billing to the patient. A standard package of benefits providing comprehensive protection against catastrophic costs would cover an estimated 156.0 million members of families with a full-time worker. Initially the NHP would limit out-of-pocket expenses for these families to $2,500 per year. All Americans would receive complete coverage (with no cost-sharing) for prenatal, delivery, and first-year care of infants. In subsequent phases the NHP would be converted into a universal, comprehensive plan by such measures as reducing cost-sharing, raising the 55 percent low-income standard, and extending fully subsidized infant care to the child's sixth year.

Under the NHP most employers are directed to purchase coverage from private insurance firms with plans certified to meet federal standards. Those employers whose premiums exceed 5 percent of payroll costs have the option of purchasing coverage from a new government-sponsored insurance fund called Healthcare at subsidized rates or of applying to Healthcare for a comparable subsidy which can be applied to private premiums. Healthcare would also cover the unemployed, the aged, the poor, and individual high-risk consumers. If NHP were enacted, employers would be required to pay at least 75 percent of the premiums. The $2,500 cap on direct payments by households would be lowered as the plan developed.

The administration's hospital cost containment plan would determine reimbursement for hospital services under the NHP. Physicians who provide services to Healthcare patients would be paid on the basis of a publicly set fee schedule based initially on Medicare statewide averages and updated through a process of negotiation between the government and physicians. Private plans would be encouraged to use this fee schedule, and the names of physicians who adhere to it would be published by the government. The NHP would also attempt to decrease the number of physicians who train for specialties now considered in oversupply, increase the number of family practitioners, and strengthen health planning in an effort to provide better health care services in medically underserved areas. The NHP would implement more rigid controls on capital expenditures, further assist in the development of health maintenance organizations (HMOs), and support preventive care and health education. The administration's plan would be financed through multiple sources—general tax revenues, premium payments by employers and employees, the Medicare payroll tax, and special excise taxes on alcohol and cigarettes.

Other Proposals

Senator Kennedy.   An alternative comprehensive national health plan with a more ambitious timetable for implementation has been proposed by Senator Kennedy. Although this plan is conceptually similar to the Carter plan, the Kennedy plan provides somewhat broader coverage and a more extensive regulatory network.

Senator Kennedy's plan would mandate universal health insurance coverage for all U.S. residents, with full coverage of inpatient hospital services, physician services in and out of hospitals, X-rays, lab tests, and some home health services. There would be no arbitrary limits on covered hospital days or physician visits under this proposal, an aspect which has the effect of providing coverage for catastrophic or major illnesses. Medicare benefits would be upgraded and would include prescription drugs.[3]

While there are many similarities between the Carter and Kennedy proposals, there are also some significant differences. First, while Carter's program would certify health plans to assure that they offer benefits consistent with those stipulated in his legislation, Kennedy's regulations regarding insurers and health plans are much more specific and stringent. In addition to mandating the insurance companies to offer a qualified health plan that includes all basic covered health care services, Kennedy's proposal specifies limitations on the number and kinds of individuals required to be enrolled in each plan and it subjects the insurance companies to ongoing review and regulation. The Kennedy proposal also stipulates that the health care records of enrolled individuals be kept by the insurers and be accessible for review by a variety of newly created regulatory entities at both state and national levels.

The primary entity of this nature would be a national health board appointed by the president to administer the Kennedy program. This board would contract with state health boards to help administer the program, and a number of commissions would be established to examine various aspects of the programs and to make recommendations to the national board.

The Kennedy plan, by adopting prospective budgeting for both hospital and physician payments for all groups of patients, would clamp relatively tighter controls on payments to providers than would the Carter bill. Under Kennedy's plan, national, state, and local budgets for health care services would place lids on health care spending, and hospital and physician charges would be prenegotiated. Insurance company premiums would be determined by negotiations between insurance companies and the government (or its national health board). Providers would negotiate with employers, unions, or the government to establish reimbursement rates and budgets and providers would not be allowed to charge patients more than is paid by an insurance plan.[4] By contrast, the Carter bill would establish physician fees only for charges to Medicare and Medicaid patients and its hospital-cost containment bill would stop short of the Kennedy proposal's full-scale prospective budgeting for hospital charges.

The financing mechanisms of the Kennedy proposal bear close resemblance to those outlined in the Carter administration's plan. Both rely heavily upon general revenues, large employer premium contributions, and Medicare payroll taxes.

Senator Long and Senators Dole, Danforth, and Domenici.   In contrast to the preceding comprehensive coverage proposals, bills introduced by Senator Long (S. 760) and Senators Dole, Danforth, and Domenici (S. 748) emphasize mandatory, employer-based, catastrophic health insurance coverage. These plans resemble the present Medicare design. Once an individual recipient or a family unit meets an out-of-pocket deductible expense for Part B—type services (drugs, doctor bills), the insurance would cover in full any further additional medical costs incurred. The size of this deductible varies according to the plan. Long's bill proposes a spending ceiling of $2,000 per year, while the Dole, Danforth, and Domenici bill allows for an initial $5,000 outlay. Both plans call for full insurance reimbursement of Part A—type services (essentially hospital services) following sixty days of hospitalization. The stop-loss provisions of both plans would confer catastrophic coverage on all workers. Senator Long's plan would assist the self-employed and low-income workers in obtaining qualified catastrophic protection. Similarly, the proposal of Senators Dole, Danforth, and Domenici provides for a residual catastrophic insurance program for people with no other insurance coverage. Benefits under both programs would be the same as those mandated under employer-based plans.

Both bills call for an expansion of Medicare and Medicaid benefits for the low-income and elderly populations. Institutional and medical copayments and benefit cutoffs would be eliminated; alternatively, the plans would reimburse the full cost of covered services when a catastrophic stop-loss trigger is reached.

The premiums for both of these catastrophic plans would be financed primarily through employer contributions, although the Dole, Danforth, and Domenici proposal relies on some government assistance. Under the Long bill, the employer could either deduct all of the premium costs as a business expense or take a 50 percent tax credit for these costs. Under the Dole bill, in contrast, if this legislation causes certain payroll costs in a taxable year to exceed 102 percent of what those costs would otherwise have been if the same level of contribution and scope of coverage had been maintained, those employers can obtain a tax credit equal to 50 percent of such excess costs in the first year after enactment, declining successively by 10 percentage points per year for each of the next four years. This provision is intended to alleviate the burden on labor-intensive employers who are likely to face larger additional costs.

Senator Durenberger.   The third group of bills, those proposed by Senators Durenberger and Schweiker and Representative Ullman, is designed to reform the health insurance system through mechanisms that differ significantly from those identified above. This group focuses upon modifications of existing financial incentives in order to encourage competition within the health care system and ultimately to gain cost containment. The hallmark of this approach to reform of the health insurance system is the fusion of employee choice of insurance plans with a system of tax incentives to encourage the selection of a low-cost plan.

In Senator Durenberger's bill, the exclusion from employees' taxable income of employer contributions to health benefits is contingent upon the element of *choice* of plans, upon a constant employer contribution to the various plans, and upon the gearing of benefit levels and federal tax breaks to national HMO standards. To qualify for federal tax breaks for health insurance contributions, employers with more than twenty-five workers must offer employees no less than three health insurance or delivery plans meeting required standards. The choice of plans includes commercial insurers and Blues (Blue Cross/Blue Shield), self-insurance, HMOs, and health and welfare funds established through collective bargaining.

Since employers must make the same contribution to all plans and since the cost (and premiums) associated with the different plans varies, employees should have an incentive to select lower-cost plans. The bill, in fact, would require that employees who select a plan in which the premium is below the employer contribution level receive the difference in taxable cash or other benefits.[5] In this way employees who select an economical package reap the savings while those who choose a more costly program pay the additional expense. Finally, the tax-free employer contribution would be limited to the nationwide average premium cost for federally qualified HMOs. Employees would have to shoulder premium costs above that cap with after-tax dollars.

The Durenberger proposal purports to reform the current system through the promotion of competition in the private sector and does not mandate *comprehensive* health insurance coverage. The plan does not call for federal financing through either payroll taxes or general revenues. It would finance the package of basic health benefits through a combination of shared premium costs and competitive incentives but—unlike some of the alternative proposals—there are no stipulations about how premium costs should be shared.

Representative Ullman.   On 30 October 1979 Representative Al Ullman introduced the Health Cost Restraint Act of 1979. The Ullman bill shares the intent of the Durenberger proposal—to encourage competition through restructuring the financing of the U.S. health care system. First, in an attempt to halt an exploding demand for health benefits, the bill imposes a limit on the tax-free premium that an employer can contribute to a health plan. A limit of $120 per month—deemed sufficient to cover comprehensive care through traditional insurance with modest deductibles and copayments or HMOs—would be placed on excludable employer contributions during the first year of the plan (1981). This limit, and other dollar figures used as cutoff points, would be updated annually in accord with increases in the Consumer Price Index.

Second, the bill requires that all employers who offer any health plan that exceeds some trigger point (e.g., $75 per month) would be subject to certain requirements in order that any of their contributions to insurance could be excluded as income by their employees.

Employees who select a plan that is more costly than the employer's $120 fixed contribution would have to pay the difference; they could keep the savings from selecting a low-option plan costing less than $120 per month. Employers would be required to offer a low-cost health plan (e.g., one costing no more than the trigger amount) with consumer cost-sharing or an HMO as alternatives to a full-benefit policy. If any plan offered exceeded the trigger cost, all options offered under that plan would have to provide a minimum level of coverage including hospital inpatient and outpatient services, physicians' services, and diagnostic, X-ray, and laboratory services. A cap of $2,000 per year (in 1981) on deductibles and copayments would be applicable to any such plan providing these services. Finally, employers must make approximately equal contributions to all options under a specific plan.

The Ullman bill briefly addresses the reform of the Medicare and Medicaid systems. It provides that an HMO be paid (prospectively) 95 percent of the costs of rendering Medicare services in the community by providers other than HMOs in order to make HMOs a viable alternative for Medicare patients. The bill also mandates a demonstration project of alternative health care delivery systems for the low-income population.

Senator Schweiker. The proposal of Senator Schweiker is very similar to the Durenberger plan, but there are a few differences worth noting. Both provide for fixed employer contributions to alternative plans with workers keeping any savings from low-cost plans. While each proposal would make tax benefits contingent upon offering workers a choice among at least three plans, only those employers with two hundred or more workers are subject to this requirement under the Schweiker plan as compared to a corresponding figure of twenty-five workers in the Durenberger plan. Under Schweiker's program, moreover, at least one of the three health plans must contain a 25 percent copayment provision for hospital charges, up to a maximum of 20 percent of family income.[6]

Another difference is that Durenberger would gear the standard benefit package to the HMO Act, while Schweiker would link the minimum required plan to the Medicare program standards plus a "preventive" package. The preventive package must contain such items as comprehensive maternal care, newborn and childhood screening for diseases, childhood immunizations, vision and hearing examinations, and hypertension screening and counseling for adults.

In addition to its focus on insurance reform in the private sector, the Schweiker plan would restructure Medicare to provide catastrophic coverage. Instead of being subject to per-hospital-spell copayments and a cutoff on the total number of hospital days covered, an individual would pay 20 percent of the cost of hospital care regardless of the cumulative number of days covered in the hospital. When the sum of Parts A and B copayments exhausts 20 percent of the patient's annual income in any one year, copayment requirements would cease.

Finally, states would be encouraged to establish a program of risk pooling which assigns to insurance companies, in proportion to the companies' business in the state, employees of small firms (less than fifty workers), uninsurable risks, and the self-employed. To assure continued involvement in federal programs, insurance companies must enroll these assigned individuals in catastrophic insurance programs. Premiums for such people could not exceed 125 percent of comparable large-group rates for similar protection in that region.

COST ESTIMATES

Estimates of the cost of national health insurance depend not only upon the scope of coverage of alternative plans, which varies widely, but also upon the perspective on costs that is selected. Some proposals would cost more than others because they would cover more people or would cover a given population more comprehensively. But for any given level of coverage in a stipulated universe it is important to distinguish on-budget federal costs for health care from total payments by individuals, and to be cognizant of the difference between the initial costs of implementing a national health insurance blueprint and the ultimate costs.

Most national health insurance proposals affect health care spending primarily by shifting the *composition* of spending or altering the *route* through which flow consumer outlays for health care. Proposals often call for new federal programs or funds, but federal outlays through these funnels typically displace some combination of federal and state spending occurring presently under existing law. In addition to affecting government outlays, most national health insurance plans would also alter federal tax revenues by changing the amount of allowable tax deductions taken by both households and firms.

It is important to recognize that NHI plans would generate substantial costs that do not appear in the federal budget. They mandate costs in the private sector that appear as line-item expenses in business budgets or, in cases where mandated costs are shared by individuals, as rising direct household outlays for health. The tendency to focus primarily on the impact on the federal budget of NHI proposals and to gloss over their impact on private spending is a specific case of the general tendency to exclusively emphasize the effect on inflation of changes in the federal budget while paying insufficient attention to the consequences of government regulation.

Initial Costs of the Carter Plan

The Carter administration's estimate of the increase in total health care spending under Phase I of the NHP (in FY 1980 dollars) is $18.3 billion over the level of systemwide outlays that would occur under current law (see Table 1).[7] This total increase is virtually identical to the projected increase in federal outlays ($18.2 billion), as the $6.1 billion increase in employer payments envisioned under Phase I is roughly offset by a decline in individual payments of $4.0 billion and a $2.0 billion drop in state payments. The bulk of the federal cost increase is attributable to improved coverage for the poor ($10.7 billion) and the aged and disabled ($3.9 billion).[8]

TABLE 1   Carter Plan Expenditures for Covered Services:
             Current Law and under NHP Phase I
             (FY 1980; amounts in billions)

	Current Law	NHP Phase I	Change
Total system spending*	$148.0	$166.3	$18.3
Federal	45.0	63.2	+18.2
Employer	42.6	48.7	+ 6.1
Individual	52.0	48.0	− 4.0
State	8.4	6.4	− 2.0

Source: U.S. Department of Health, Education and Welfare, *Fact Sheet* (Washington, DC), 12 June 1979, p. 35.
   *For NHP covered services.

The Growth of Costs under the Carter Plan

Increased coverage. In assessing projections of future costs of NHI, it is useful to begin with the greater program costs that will emerge from planned benefit enrichments and more widespread coverage. First, the plan envisions ultimately covering all of the poor, whereas in Phase I only those with incomes below 55 percent of the poverty line will be automatically covered. In view of the estimate by the Department of Health, Education, and Welfare (HEW) that it will cost $5.5 billion to cover those below the 55 percent threshold and the likelihood that there are fewer people in this group than there are in the non-Medicaid poor group between the threshold and the poverty line, the cost of filling that gap would probably exceed $5.5 billion. Indeed, HEW estimates that it would cost $3.8 billion to cover in Phase I that portion of the poverty group above the threshold who "spend down" to the threshold. If this estimate assumes that about one of four households eligible for this spend-down provision use it and that it would cost about the same per household to cover those who do not, a rough estimate of $15−16 billion (in 1980 dollars) emerges for covering the whole group between the 55 percent threshold and the poverty line.

Second, the plan envisions extending and enriching the employer guarantee. Part-time workers are ultimately to be included, and it is reasonable to assume that this will add at least $1.0 billion to employer costs.[9] And according to the administration's proposal: "Cost-sharing could be reduced and deductibles eliminated, converting catastropic coverage to comprehensive coverage." (HEW 1979, p. 40). This, of course, initially represents only a transfer of costs from households to employers, but it could ultimately increase total outlays if consumers are induced to use more health services when they face a smaller cost restraint.

There are several other areas in which the HEW plan contemplates broader benefits during subsequent phases of NHI. First, cost-sharing would be reduced for the aged and disabled who would also begin to receive drug benefits. Second, the plan would ultimately extend the prenatal, delivery, and infant benefits through the child's sixth year without patient cost-sharing. Third, comprehensive coverage could be required for people outside of the labor force who are neither poor nor aged. Such people would have the option in Phase I of "buying into" the Healthcare fund. This group would include people who are spouses of Medicare recipients but are not eligible themselves, disabled people for whom a mandatory disability-benefit waiting period has not elapsed, and single people who are not in the work force but who have sufficient income from nonworking sources to be above the poverty level. Finally, administrative costs and tax effects will change as the coverage and comprehensiveness of the program change. At the present time there are no cost estimates available for these proposed benefit changes, but they would clearly add to the out-year costs of NHI.

Offsets from Cost Containment

The Carter administration expects to offset cost increases emerging from its NHI proposal with cost controls and changes in the health care system.

Reductions from cost controls and system reform incentives are estimated to more than offset the expanded utilization and expenditures generated by the Phase I plan after the third year of operation. Even with the expansion to the fully implemented universal, comprehensive plan, total health spending is expected to be lower than it would be under the current system. [HEW 1979, p. 35]

There are several reasons why these expectations are unlikely to be fulfilled. First, the hospital cost containment legislation, a mainstay of the administration's plan to control cost increases, has not been enacted by Congress though it has been under consideration for over two years.[10]

Second, the particular form of the current proposal seems to be so riddled with exclusions, exceptions, and contingencies as to make it unlikely that it would have any bite. Three triggers must go off before any hospital can possibly be in jeopardy. Labor costs, now accounting for about 50 percent of total costs for the average hospital, are in effect exempted from the cap. There are numerous ways in which hospitals could unbundle services or spin off functions to evade the intent of the proposal. There also is wide latitude for HEW to grant special adjustments or exemptions for various special circumstances.

Third, even with more bite, the proposal would seem capable of producing only short-term results and some of these results would be likely to take the form of undesired service cutbacks or quality reductions. Since the system of financial incentives and reimbursement mechanisms would essentially remain unchanged, there is little reason to believe that the legislation would spur hospitals to eliminate inefficiencies rather than to redefine, relocate, or simply cut services.

Congressional Budget Office (CBO) estimates of the savings arising from the proposed 1979 Hospital Cost Containment Act are considerably lower than the administration's estimates. CBO's estimated reduction in annual hospital inpatient revenues in fiscal year 1980 is $1.2 billion,[11] as compared to the administration's estimated savings of $2.3 billion. The corresponding figures for FY 1984 are $11.3 billion and $19.2 billion. (CBO 1979a, pp 29–38).[12] The last figure—the administration's estimate of 1984 savings from cost containment—roughly corresponds with the estimated NHI cost for the first year in which the plan would be implemented ($18.3 billion in FY 1983), explaining the administration's contention that the two bills would offset each other from a cost viewpoint. But the CBO figure of $11.3 billion suggests that this contention is overly optimistic.[13]

Finally, even if the administration's estimate of cost containment savings is accepted for the first or second year of NHI implementation, it is highly unlikely that any ongoing savings would fully offset the swelling cost of NHI in its subsequent phases. Furthermore, to the extent that many hospitals "comply" with cost containment by cutting services or slowing quality improvements, we would, curiously, be "financing" NHI's health benefit improvements for some consumers through cutbacks in the benefits for others. Indeed, some consumers may obtain improved insurance coverage (with more services reimbursed) at lower cost, but receive a style of hospital care that falls short of the desired treatment.

The administration's plan would also contain health care costs through "negotiations" with doctors to update allowable physicians' fees for doctors who serve people covered by Healthcare. Negotiations over allowable fee schedules could be expected to degenerate into a test of political strength, and it is by no means clear that the government will have the bargaining strength to achieve its targets. By clamping a lid on allowable charges to Healthcare patients, moreover, the government may inadvertently foster a situation in which these patients have relatively less access to high quality services performed in a timely fashion.

In addition to savings arising from the proposed hospital cost containment bill, the administration's plan envisions savings from "incentive effects." But such favorable effects regrettably are likely to be limited under the scenario envisioned by the Carter proposal. The NHP's answer to a lack of consumer choice among alternative delivery systems—an important cause of health-care cost escalation (Enthoven 1979) — is further government stimulus to HMOs. This would be done through such means as requiring employers of twenty-five or more workers to offer their employees a choice between an insurance plan and all participating HMOs in the area. Federal efforts to stimulate in this fashion the growth of HMOs as alternatives to traditional fee-for-service health care delivery have not met with much success since the passage of the 1973 HMO legislation.[14] Requirements that HMOs maintain standards of comprehensiveness which in some cases exceed those typical of private health insurance policies, along with preferences by many consumers for a fee-for-service arrangement, have limited the development of HMOs. More important, the president's NHP proposal offers little incentive for a *variety* of health delivery models—including those which differ in some respect from either classical HMOs or traditional fee-for-service models—to develop and compete.[15]

Moreover, the Carter proposal would solidify the current job-centered nature of most insurance purchases in which employers provide their workers with either a single insurance package or the choice between a standard package of benefits and an HMO. The administration's insistence, in the name of administrative simplicity and equity, on a standard minimum benefit package throughout the private economy tends to make the choice of insurance—one place in the health care area where the consumer clearly *could* have control over health expenditures—a rigid one. The proposal would permit employees to obtain the savings from selecting a lower-cost plan, and this is a step in the right direction. But the favorable impact of this feature is limited by the fact that plans must provide all of the benefits stipulated in the proposed bill; this will place a (rather high) floor on costs and thereby limit possible savings. It is essential to provide people with a meaningful choice among various health packages (not just the streamlined HMO alternative) with very different combinations of benefits, premiums, and cost-sharing, and to ensure that consumers benefit from the selection of a relatively low-cost option. One of the reasons why the cost of the administration's NHI proposal is likely to balloon over time is that it is not apt to stimulate such competition effectively; indeed it may unintentionally retard it due to an emphasis on a standard benefit package rather than on a variegated set of alternatives.

It is worth noting, by contrast, that the bill allows for copayments up to a maximum of $2,500 per year, and this should act as a deterrent to the overconsumption of health services. This advantage may dwindle over time, however, as the plan envisions scaling down the cap on household copayments.

Other Proposals

The Kennedy plan has somewhat broader coverage than the Carter bill, as is reflected in the figure for total U.S. spending (in 1980 dollars) for health services covered by Kennedy's plan—

TABLE 2
Comparative Summary of Major NHI Proposals[a]

Benefit Categories	Proposal Sponsors and Program Provisions	Initial Annual Cost (Expenditures)[b]
Mandatory comprehensive benefits	Kennedy (S. 1720)	
	Comprehensive coverage, all health care services	$40[c]
	Extensive regulatory network: negotiate and establish reimbursement rates for hospitals, physicians, insurance plans, federal and state program administration	
	Financing: employer contributions, general revenue, Medicare payroll tax	
	Carter (S. 1812)	
	Phase-in comprehensive benefits	$18[d]
	Phase I: mandatory standard benefit package, including catastrophic	
	Cost sharing for Medicare recipients and working families	
	Comprehensive coverage for prenatal and first year care	
	Influence supply of physicians and control reimbursement rates	
	Financing: employer and employee contributions, Medicare payroll tax; general tax revenues; special excise taxes	
Mandatory catastrophic benefits	Long (S. 760) and Dole, Danforth, and Domenici (S. 748)[e]	$6-7[f]
	Full payment of all medical costs incurred after recipient meets substantial out-of-pocket deductible	
	Expansion of Medicaid and Medicare benefits	
	Financing: employer contributions, minimum government assistance	

Benefit Categories	Proposal Sponsors and Program Provisions	Initial Annual Cost (Expenditures)[b]

Tax incentives to stimulate competition	Durenberger (S. 1968)
	Employer contributions tax deductible if:
	  Employer offers employees choice of health insurance plans
	  Uniform employer contribution to plans
	  Benefit and cost levels modeled on HMO standards
	  Employee saves or pays for plans chosen
		$—[g]

	Ullman (H.R. 5740) Employer provisions (tax-break contingencies) same as Durenberger, and provides for Medicare reimbursement for HMO enrollment	$—

	Schweiker (S. 1590)
	  Employer provisions same as in Durenberger plan for employers with more than 200 employees
	  Pooled risks programs for employees in small firms
	  Medicare coverage of catastrophic illnesses
	  Minimum benefit package modeled after Medicare standards and includes preventive coverage
		$3.8

[a]This summary is provided to assist the reader in comparing the broad, conceptual approaches to the NHI issue. The specific provisions of each bill and the individual cost estimates are, of course, subject to considerable change as the legislative debate over NHI unfolds.

[b]FY 1980; amounts in billions. Represents increases in total health care spending.

[c]On-budget federal outlays account for $28.6 billion of this total figure, while the $11.4 billion balance represents increased employer outlays.

[d]As Carter's plan is phased-in, benefits and coverage will increase as cost-sharing phases down. The ultimate expenditures, therefore, should approach those estimates for the Kennedy plan.

[e]The Subcommittee on Health of the Senate Finance Committee is currently incorporating features of both bills into a single, modified proposal.

[f]This figure represents initial rough estimates for proposed catastrophic plans; if, however, a bill emerges from the Senate Finance Committee which also incorporates some of the low income benefits included in more comprehensive proposals, the price tag for such legislation would rise sharply. It is also important to note that any initial cost estimates for catastrophic plans have significant growth potential as covered benefits increase.

[g]Under the Durenberger and Ullman plans, the federal government is not expected to increase budget outlays, and it may realize additional tax revenues.

$171.4 billion. The corresponding figure for the Carter plan is
$148.0 billion. If the Kennedy plan were implemented in FY
1983, total spending for covered services would rise to an estimated $211.4 billion (in 1980 dollars), representing a projected
total program cost of $40 billion for the first year[16] as compared
to the figure of $18.3 billion for the Carter plan. Much of the
difference, of course, represents the phasing of the Carter proposal rather than major differences in ultimate coverage. Of the
$40 billion initial cost of the Kennedy program, $28.6 billion
would be accounted for by rising on-budget federal costs (i.e.,
federal outlays would total $79.6 billion in 1983 under the Ken-
nedy plan instead of the projected $51.0 billion for the same
covered services under current law).

Senator Schweiker's Comprehensive Health Reform Plan carries a smaller price tag than the Carter and Kennedy proposals.
Schweiker estimates that his bill will result in a savings in
systemwide health outlays of $3.7 billion in the first year, but
this figure includes projected savings of $7.5 billion from a hos-
pital cost containment bill. Without such a bill the Schweiker
plan per se is projected to increase outlays by $3.8 billion.

It is worth noting that a little more than half of this estimated
increase in outlays is attributed to the cost of Schweiker's mandated preventive health program ($2.0 billion), and this figure
does not include any offset for savings due to lower expenses required to treat illnesses diagnosed early and for a reduction in
lost output and earnings from worker illness. The remainder of
the increase in outlays is accounted for by the cost of Medicare
improvements ($0.8 billion) and the cost of the catastrophic ill-
ness pooling program for employees of small firms, high-risk
uninsured individuals, and the self-employed ($1.0 billion).

Furthermore, unlike the Carter and Kennedy plans, this proposal would take steps in the direction of modifying tax incentives and stimulating broad choices among competing health
plans, two changes that are vital to the achievement of lasting
moderation in cost escalation.

THE PROBLEM WITH THE CARTER
AND KENNEDY PROPOSALS

With either the Carter or Kennedy proposals, the ultimate impact on costs will hinge on the capacity of their constraints on providers for permanently limiting cost increases. Neither proposal would significantly alter the structural forces stimulating demand, while both would intensify the upward pressure on demand by broadening insurance coverage and making it more comprehensive. This upward pressure is to be "contained" by controls on charges and by the anticipated challenge from federally qualified HMOs.

The problem with these proposals is not that they aim to extend insurance coverage to millions of Americans who currently lack coverage or that they seek to remove various limitations on the coverage that others currently maintain. Whether we want to ensure that all Americans have a comprehensive package of insurance benefits is an important policy question, but its answer will only be a first step in evaluating the impact of NHI on private health care costs and the federal budget. The ultimate cost of guaranteeing a minimum insurance package to everyone would depend on how this guarantee is financed and on the mechanisms established to discourage wasteful spending on health care.

Assuming the premise that such waste emanates largely from the providers' control over patients and from their desire to increase earnings or profits by overtesting and overhospitalizing unwary patients, the Carter and Kennedy proposals would attempt to finance NHI through a squeeze on providers. This squeeze is likely to be counterproductive, leading either to greater cost acceleration or to cuts in services while the fundamental forces leading to waste—inextricably involved with the growth and current nature of insurance—are left largely unaltered.

The argument over the Carter and Kennedy proposals is, in a sense, a microcosm of the controversy over government attempts to clamp economywide controls on suppliers while simultaneously stimulating demand in the overall economy. And the result—rapid cost and price increases, shortages, and quality problems—is likely to be the same. Past attempts to increase the rate of growth in a nation's money supply above the pace that would otherwise be considered prudent, relying on wage and price controls to ensure that this excessive growth improves real variables such as production and employment without accelerating inflation, have typically resulted in various supply shortfalls and black markets and ultimately caused a spurt in inflation as controls are relaxed.

Similarly, if the demand for health services is stimulated through substantial increases in the depth and breadth of insurance coverage while supply is constrained through controls on hospital beds and charges as well as on physician supply and fees, the result will tend to be a combination of longer waiting times for treatment, a deterioration in the quality of service, and an explosion in costs when consumers ultimately insist on a restoration of the kind of services to which they had grown accustomed.

The Carter and Kennedy proposals would convert the carrot of open-ended tax breaks (designed to encourage comprehensive insurance) into a mandate; yet they would leave the tax breaks intact, failing even to convert them into fixed-dollar credits that would limit their yield. Thus everyone would receive automatically what the government deems to be minimal insurance protection and would be rewarded for doing so through tax incentives that become a kind of windfall. And the proposals forego an opportunity to encourage meaningful competition among a variety of alternative delivery systems by taking a "uniform package" approach rather than by stimulating the kind of heterogeneous insurance environment in which consumers can select the mix of benefits, costs, and risks that suits their own tastes.

Of course, the aim of these proposals is not simply to control health care cost increases; their primary goal is to assure access to care for all U.S. citizens irrespective of age and income. But both proposals suggest that this assurance can be given *without* a major long-term impact on costs by use of a system of strict provider controls, and it is this pledge that is misleading. If we are going to insure everyone and to remove the cost consequences of major illness, we are going to have to pay for it. Through an elaborate system of provider controls it may be possible to mask or divert temporarily some of this cost from a monetary to a nonmonetary form, but we cannot make the cost evaporate.

Efforts to freeze the share of gross national product (GNP) accounted for by health care expenditures through negotiating or legislating "acceptable" fees and charges seem to fly in the face of free consumer choices. It would be more prudent to alter those forces that distort consumer choice and feed wasteful spending so that such growth as occurs in the health care share of GNP is simply a sign of consumer preference for more health care—in return for which the consumer is willing to sacrifice some other goods and services. Surely we do not want to freeze permanently the shares of the economic pie accounted for by food, health, housing, etc.

Housing costs have also been rising as a share of GNP, and we provide open-ended subsidies for a significant portion of the cost of owner-occupied housing. Are we to cap this growth by controls on home builders?

There is growing evidence, both from studies of controls on hospitals[17] and from general evaluations of cost-plus regulatory interventions, that a regulatory approach to cost containment will not provide the anticipated results. Indeed, the increasingly complex body of federal and state regulations is beginning to be viewed as much as a *part* of the health cost problem as it is a *cure*. Given this mounting evidence, it becomes important that we think carefully about the need for a new federal program in this area. Surely there has been a problem of underinsurance in the United States, and this problem needs to be addressed. But to what extent is this problem disappearing as people become more aware of the availability of low-cost catastrophic insurance? To what extent could those people who fall between the cracks of public and private insurance be helped by modifications in current programs (e.g., reform of Medicaid and Medicare) or through the establishment of a pooled-risk fund to serve those otherwise deemed uninsurable? Do we need a national program, with universal mandated minimum coverage, in order to solve this problem of underinsurance?

If we do strive to solve the problem through a new federal program, it will be important to evaluate alternative proposals in terms of their provisions for eliminating both underinsurance and the concomitant problem of overinsurance. In this regard it is important that an effort to increase insurance coverage, if undertaken, be accompanied by structural modifications that hold more promise for a lasting abatement of wasteful spending.

9

KEITH B. LEFFLER

COTTON M. LINDSAY

The Long-Run Effects of National Health Insurance on Medical Care Prices and Output*

The escalation of medical costs under NHI. Three alternative plans. Patient demand and the supply of physicians—the danger of shortages. Price controls in the medical market; their effect on medical schools. Economic losses due to queue rationing.

*Reprinted from original 1976 study. No new developments invalidate the findings published at that time.

One of the most dramatic effects of the increased governmental role in providing for medical care is rapid escalation of physician fees and hospital prices.[1] This results from a drastic increase in demand for a relatively fixed supply of medical services. Table 1 illustrates the price escalation from Medicare. Overall medical care prices increased 51 percent faster than the general price index in a five-year period after the implementation of Medicare. Total real expenditures on health care rose by 42 percent, but the relative increased price of medical care accounted for nearly

TABLE 1   Health and Medical Care Expenditures and Prices 1965, 1970, 1973[a]

	1965	1970	1973
Total Expenditures	38,892	68,083	94,070
Total Expenditures			
1965 dollars (CPI deflated)	38,892	55,352	66,811
1965 dollars (Medical Care Index deflated)	38,892	50,544	61,164
Public Expenditures	9,529	25,259	37,534
Percent of total	24.5	37.1	39.9
Hospital Care			
Total	13,152	25,895	36,200
Public	4,930	12,931	19,249
Public share	37.5	49.9	53.2
Physician Services			
Total	8,405	13,450	18,040
Public	527	3,120	4,041
Public share	6.3	23.2	22.4
Consumer Price Index	100.0	123.0	140.8
Medical Care Price Index	100.0	134.7	153.8
Hospital Care[b] Price Index	100.0	191.6	239.9
Physician Services Price Index	100.0	137.5	156.5

[a]All amounts in millions of dollars.

[b]Includes only semi-private room rates.

Source: All expenditure data, U.S. Department of Health, Education, and Welfare; all price data, U S. Department of Labor.

a third of this increase. Expenditures for physician services rose 60 percent while the quantity supplied only rose 16 percent. We have estimated that by the end of 1967 Medicare caused a $7,000 increase in the gross income of an average physician in private practice (Leffler 1977, Chapter 2; Lindsay et al. 1976, Chapter 3).

The effect on hospital bed prices is even more dramatic, as the price nearly doubled in the five-year period following the adoption of Medicare. In late 1971 the health care sector of the economy was constrained by wage and price controls; since then the impact of Medicare on prices has been difficult to assess. However, the public share of medical care spending has risen by only 2 percent annually since 1971, which suggests that the impact of these programs already may have peaked. At any rate, medical care price inflation has only kept pace with general price rises since 1970.

National health insurance (NHI) will increase the demand for all forms of medical care. We predict, however, that it will have its greatest impact on the demand for physicians' services and drugs. NHI will influence prices by lowering the cost to consumers of increased consumption of medical care, thereby encouraging increased demand. Since third parties (private insurance companies and federal, state, and local governments) already pay over 90 percent of expenditures for hospital care, the scope of reduced costs for hospitals is relatively slight. In the hospital sector NHI will therefore have the principal effect of rerouting these payments through the federal government rather than through private insurers and nonfederal governments. This is not to argue that such a change would be inconsequential, however. A 1975 General Accounting Office (GAO) study of the Social Security Administration's performance in reimbursing providers found that it costs the government nearly twice what it costs private insurers to process Medicare claims. (GAO 1975).

Under NHI the demand for drugs and prescriptions might increase greatly. In 1973 consumers personally paid over 85 percent of their drug expenditures. The various proposed insurance schemes differ in their treatment of drugs, some including deductibles and copayment; but all would stimulate demand to some extent. The impact of insurance on drug prices would nevertheless be negligible because the response of supply in the drug industry is rapid and output expansion historically has had little lasting effect on costs of production (see Cocks and Virts 1974). From 1965 to 1970, in fact, drug prescription prices fell by 16 percent relative to the general price index.

If NHI is adopted, major price escalation can be predicted for physician services. Consumers now pay over 40 percent of their medical expenditures for physician services. Private insurance payments account for an additional 36 percent. Several of the proposed plans, including the Corman-Kennedy bill and the Javits bill, provide unlimited payments for physician services with minor or no copayments or deductibles. However, unlike the pharmaceutical industry, the supply of physicians can adjust only very gradually to changes in demand. A large increase in demand for their services would therefore stimulate significant and lasting price increases unless and until the supply of physicians expanded.

Because of limited predicted effects of NHI on hospital and drug prices, this chapter will focus on the predicted impact of national health insurance on physician fees and earnings. The discussion may be conveniently divided into two sections. First we will report results of an aggregative long-run model of the market for physician services in which we simulate conditions under various assumptions about the extent of insurance provided. The model's predictions concerning annual prices and numbers of physicians under these various assumptions are reported through the year 2000.

NHI proposals often include plans to control prices by government fiat, however. For example, the Corman-Kennedy 1974 proposals contain stringent cost control measures emphasizing capitation and salary reimbursement even for physicians in solo practice. The second part of the chapter will predict the effects of such price controls superimposed by various possible insurance programs. Our model directly estimates the effects of price controls on future physician supply, and we have attempted at the end of the section crudely to quantify the social costs of such controls.

PRICES AND QUANTITIES WITHOUT CONTROLS

Figure 1 illustrates the basic design of our model of the market for physician services. The private market for physician services is influenced by population levels and income. National health insurance also operates on the demand side of the market by lowering the effective price which consumers must pay for care. The question is how much will it lower the price? As an index of this price discount we use the percentage of expenditures paid by third parties. We will examine three alternatives. The first we will assume (Plan A) is taken to be no national health insurance. The average consumer will pay a declining percentage of expenditures (computed at the trend rate) because of increased utilization of private health insurance and an increasing percentage of the aged covered by Medicare. Table 2, column A, shows the assumed percentage of direct consumer payments from 1976 to 2000.

Plan B is intended to represent a "moderate" national health insurance plan—which may be thought of as an extension of a Medicare-type plan to the poorer segments of the population. Such a plan has the essential characteristics of the Medical Expense Tax Credit Act introduced by Senator William Brock and of the Long-Ribicoff proposals. This plan is assumed to extend gradually and be implemented over a five-year period, as shown in column B of Table 2.

The third alternative, Plan C, is taken to involve complete coverage of physician fees in the manner of the Corman-Kennedy bill or the Medicredit plan endorsed by the American

FIGURE 1
A MODEL OF THE MARKET FOR PHYSICIAN SERVICES

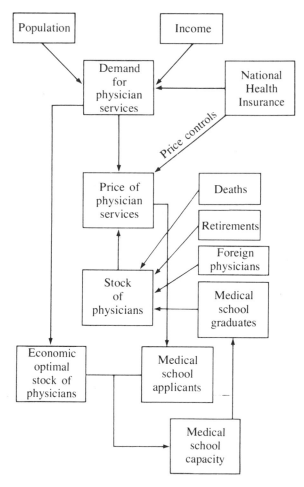

TABLE 2   Assumed Impact of Various National
Health Insurance Schemes

Percentage of Expenditures on Physician Services
by Direct Consumer Repayment

	A No NHI	B Moderate Plan	C Plan Complete
1976	39	39	39
1977	38	35	1
1978	37	30	1
1979	36	25	1
1980	35	20	1
1981	34	15	1
1982	33	10	1
1983	32	10	1
1984	31	10	1
1985	30	10	1
1986	29	10	1
1987	28	10	1
1988	27	10	1
1989	26	10	1
1990	25	10	1
1991	25	10	1
1992	25	10	1
1993	25	10	1
1994	25	10	1
1995	25	10	1
1996	25	10	1
1997	25	10	1
1998	25	10	1
1999	25	10	1
2000	25	10	1

Medical Association. The full plan is assumed to impact on the economy rapidly, with full implementation during 1977. Column C of Table 2 shows the assumed percentage of physician services expenditures made directly by consumers under this plan.

Given these assumptions about the demand side of the market and the modeling of supply behavior developed below, we may reasonably predict prices and quantities of physician services over the next twenty-five years. Economists have argued, however, that the classic market-pricing model may not be applicable to physician-pricing decisions (see Feldstein 1970b). Physicians may trade off interesting and novel cases for increased fees, thereby creating a continual excess demand. This sort of behavior poses no problem for our model as long as "desired" excess demand is related to total demand in a stable manner.[2]

The appendix to the chapter describes eight equations in our model of the market for physician services with supporting discussion. The equations have all been estimated using data from 1947 to 1973. We shall restrict ourselves here to briefly outlining the structure of the model.

At a given point in time the supply of services is essentially fixed by the stock of physicians. Minor supply increases might result from movements of research physicians into primary-care activities as well as increased work hours from retired or semi-retired physicians. Assuming that supply in any one period is perfectly unresponsive to price, we should be able to predict price at any time on the basis of supply and demand related variables. In fact, such an equation explains more than 98 percent of the variance in physician earnings—and therefore presumably fees—during the period considered.

For such a price equation to be useful, however, both the stock of physicians and these demand variables themselves must be predicted for future periods. Demand variables were simply extrapolated from past trends; however, we felt that economic theory could provide a better framework for predicting the number of physicians in any year. In the period following adoption of the Medicare-Medicaid legislation, the output rate of physicians (and ultimately the stock) in any period was surprisingly sensitive to economic variables as capacity of medical schools increased over 65 percent from 1966 to 1974.

Returning to Figure 1, we observe four influences on the stock of physicians: deaths, retirements, emigration, and new medical graduates. Deaths and retirements are estimated from a constant percentage of last years' stock. Emigration is assumed to be determined by the size of the existing "shortage" of physicians. Graduates of medical schools may be constrained by two influences. On the one hand, clearly the number of locally trained physicians is limited by the capacity of American medical schools. Hall (1976a) has shown that medical school capacity experiences a lag in adjusting to the socially desired stock of physicians—which stock is defined as that level of practitioners which yields them no monopoly return.

On the other hand, medical schools are limited by the number of qualified applicants. Society imposes quality standards on those who practice medicine, and these standards are enforced on medical school graduates by state licensing boards. The historical ratios of medical school applicants to acceptances are quite stable in periods without monopoly returns, which suggests that never more than one-half of all medical school applicants have sufficient ability to succeed in school and pass licensing standards.[3]

The total number of applicants itself has been shown to be related to the expected relative attractiveness of a medical career. Leffler (1977)[4] has estimated this relationship (between attractiveness and applicant numbers) and has found he can explain more than 97 percent of the variance in the applicant rate on the basis of the pecuniary attractiveness of the medical career. This result is reproduced as equation 3 in the appendix.

Supply behavior may then be summarized as follows: medical school capacity is projected on the basis of a lag in adjustment to what is predicted to be the socially desired stock of physicians, given the level of other parameters in the system. However, the ability of medical schools to train physicians is constrained by the availability of qualified applicants. Often it is the supply of qualified applicants rather than medical school capacity which limits the output of new physicians. This is particularly important in weighing the effects and merits of price controls. Data presented below indicate that price controls in an extensive health insurance scheme such as the Corman-Kennedy bill will reduce the number of qualified applicants and thereby constrain medical school outputs—severely impairing what might otherwise be a reasonably rapid adjustment to this (i.e., NHI) market intervention.

Table 3 presents our estimates of the effects of three alternative plans on physician fees and earnings. These predictions are in current dollars and apply to the median general practitioner in solo practice. In the absence of national health insurance, physician fees are expected to rise at an average annual rate of slightly less than 1.5 percent. Earnings over the period should increase from the 1976 level of $45,169 to $65,686 by the year 2000. The next four years (1976–1980) should continue the real decline of the last four as strong adjustment continues to the demand increase generated by the Medicare program. The overall general rise over the rest of this century results in the main from increased earnings throughout the economy. In order to attract qualified college graduates into medical training, the earnings of physicians must keep pace with those throughout the economy. Our model assumes that the median college graduate's earnings will rise from $16,129 in 1976 to $27,530 by 2000, representing an average growth rate of 2 percent.

The moderate insurance plan is assumed to be implemented gradually. Its immediate effect should be small. Increased demand will tend to offset the otherwise downward adjustment towards equilibrium. Average physician fees are predicted to rise from $9.32 in 1976 to $10.93 by 1980. By 1982, however, when the moderate plan is fully implemented, physician fees will have risen by 42 percent. At that time physician earnings

TABLE 3   Estimated Physician Fees and Earnings under Three
            Alternative NHI Plans, 1976–2000

	No NHI Earnings[1]	No NHI Fee[2]	Moderate NHI Earnings[1]	Moderate NHI Fee[2]	Complete NHI Earnings[1]	Complete NHI Fee[2]
1976	44,748	9.32	44,748	9.32	44,748	9.32
1977	44,021	9.17	45,380	9.45	168,870	35.18
1978	43,443	9.05	47,054	9.80	165,401	34.46
1979	43,405	9.04	49,405	10.29	158,030	32.92
1980	43,762	9.12	52,479	10.93	151,027	31.46
1981	44,378	9.25	56,714	11.82	144,371	30.08
1982	45,218	9.42	63,521	13.23	138,270	28.81
1983	46,141	9.61	60,884	12.68	132,676	27.64
1984	47,152	9.82	58,466	12.18	127,545	26.57
1985	48,257	10.05	56,249	11.72	121,763	25.37
1986	49,463	10.30	54,387	11.33	115,422	24.05
1987	50,775	10.58	53,489	11.14	108,620	22.63
1988	52,204	10.88	53,404	11.13	101,699	21.19
1989	53,757	11.20	53,823	11.21	94,943	19.78
1990	55,447	11.55	54,461	11.35	88,574	18.45
1991	56,383	11.75	55,185	11.50	82,712	17.23
1992	57,253	11.93	55,865	11.64	77,394	16.12
1993	58,240	12.13	56,470	11.76	72,587	15.12
1994	59,343	12.36	57,032	11.88	68,236	14.22
1995	60,447	12.59	57,581	12.00	64,291	13.39
1996	61,538	12.82	58,141	12.11	61,916	12.90
1997	62,607	13.04	58,725	12.23	60,939	12.70
1998	63,649	13.26	59,341	12.36	60,778	12.66
1999	64,673	13.47	59,988	12.50	60,636	12.63
2000	65,686	13.68	60,663	12.64	60,504	12.61

[1]Median net earnings before tax, solo general practitioners (1975 dollars).

[2]Median fee for an office visit to a solo general practitioner in private practice (1975 dollars).

203

are predicted to be $63,521, which implies that physicians will be receiving $18,739 per year more than is required to make medicine an attractive career.

Figure 2 illustrates an interesting characteristic of this market. From 1990 until 2000 our model predicts the equilibrium fees under the moderate insurance plan will be lower than would exist if no NHI was instituted. This result is predicted because of an expected overshooting response to shortages in this and other human capital training markets.[5] This is likely to occur because both schools and applicants tend to respond to variables which lag as much as eight years behind by rapid increases in demand: thus, when the supply does finally respond, it tends to overrespond. The shock of demand from Medicare produced exactly this effect. Our predicted fees without NHI over the career of physicians who are just now entering medical school are inadequate to cover the costs of medical training. Entering physicians thus are expected to earn a severe net loss of their investment in training. However, the number of applicants to medical schools is growing and will continue to grow for several years because fees are just now beginning to fall. This market overshooting in response to the Medicare program of the previous decade may serve to mitigate the initial demand shock resulting from adoption of a national health insurance plan.

The impact of a complete national health insurance plan is more tenuously predicted. Our estimating equations were very robust in explaining data up to 1973 and we believe they are quite accurate for predictions based on past experience. A complete insurance scheme is not such an event; rather it will produce a demand shock in a single-year period equivalent to demand changes occurring over the prior thirty years. Nonetheless, our estimates provide a rough guide to the order of magnitude of price increases to be expected. Figure 2 indicates the magnitude and severity of the demand shock on the physician service market engendered by a complete national health insurance scheme. The median market-clearing fee in the first year of the complete program would be about $35, nearly a four-

FIGURE 2
PHYSICIAN FEES

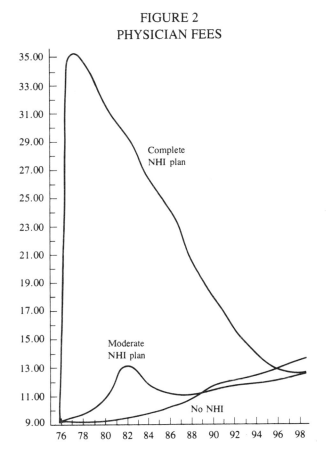

TABLE 4   Estimated Stock of Physicians and Physician
Shortages under Two NHI Plans 1976–2000

	Moderate Plan Estimated Stock Shortage[1]		Complete Plan Estimated Stock Shortage		No Plan Estimated Stock Shortage	
1976	407,729	23,100	407,729	23,100	407,729	23,100
1977	423,061	21,595	423,061	245,760	423,061	16,410
1978	435,965	23,890	435,965	283,336	435,965	10,268
1979	448,570	28,334	453,171	226,683	447,666	6,246
1980	461,834	34,767	470,394	215,088	457,538	3,778
1981	476,290	44,151	487,638	203,546	466,537	2,309
1982	492,138	59,644	504,624	192,336	474,840	1,665
1983	509,056	48,577	521,355	181,457	483,018	1,279
1984	525,721	37,840	537,835	170,904	491,073	1,153
1985	542,136	27,428	555,568	159,175	499,008	1,289
1986	557,764	17,879	574,578	146,243	506,823	1,690
1987	570,555	11,243	594,893	132,084	514,521	2,360
1988	580,851	7,182	616,146	117,065	522,104	3,304
1989	589,612	4,731	637,965	101,556	529,573	4,525
1990	597,763	2,969	659,973	85,938	536,930	6,030
1991	605,743	1,458	681,888	70,491	544,308	5,121
1992	613,959	−210	703,529	55,398	551,999	3,977
1993	622,499	−2,124	724,845	40,708	559,460	3,142
1994	631,260	−4,177	745,841	26,420	566,711	2,599
1995	640,149	−6,278	766,523	12,527	574,091	2,008
1996	649,097	−8,356	783,543	2,377	581,638	1,331
1997	658,064	−10,371	796,930	−4,058	589,374	548
1998	667,035	−12,307	808,133	−8,226	597,306	−350
1999	676,011	−14,165	819,357	−12,333	605,412	−1,338
2000	685,006	−15,958	830,632	−16,405	613,663	−2,386

[1]Derived by subtracting the estimated stock from the stock which would yield zero economic rent—that is, just pay for the physician's training investment. The zero rent stocks are given in the appendix.

fold increase over the prior year. Physician earnings would peak that first year at over $168,000. Once again, with some overshooting, by the year 2000 fees would be lowest under the complete plan.

Table 4 shows the estimated stock of physicians under the three alternative plans. Because of lags in adjustment there is no predicted difference in stocks until 1979. From then on, however, the supply of physicians under the complete and moderate plans should increase relative to the stock if no plan is instituted.

Table 4 also gives the physician shortage until the twenty-first century. By shortage here we do not mean that, at the predicted prices, the market for physicians does not clear. On the contrary, the model assumes perfect flexibility of prices in the short run. We use shortage in the alternative "human capital" sense of indicating a difference in the existing stock of physicians and that which would prevail in the long run under static demand conditions. Shortages do not occur in the usual economic sense. In the absence of externally imposed impediments such as price controls, prices will rise until the total amount demanded will equal the total amount supplied. Thus we say that markets "clear," with price being the variable that adjusts to the clearing level. As was pointed out above, both medical schools and students make their decisions on the basis of previous years' information. This implies that, given changing economic conditions, earnings are rarely at the level expected by physicians when they made the decision to enter medical school. Thus the number is rarely that which would exist if their expectations had been correct.[6]

With no national health insurance plan, we note that the shortages created by the adoption of the Medicare-Medicaid programs in the mid-1960s are even today rapidly disappearing. By 1980 such shortages are negligible, i.e., less than 1 percent of the physician force. For the gradually introduced moderate plan, the shortage peaks at the same time that coverage reaches its maximum level in 1982. The shortage at this time is 59,644 or

12 percent of the stock. Ten years later, in 1992, the market should have fully adjusted. Some overshooting follows, as indicated by a physician surplus of about 2 percent in the year 2000. For the complete plan, the shortage is much more severe and immediate. In the first year of the plan we predict a physician shortage of 58 percent representing 248,760 physicians. The time required to reach equilibrium is also longer, with full adjustment not expected until twenty years after the plan is instituted. Once again a surplus is predicted in the year 2000.

FIGURE 3

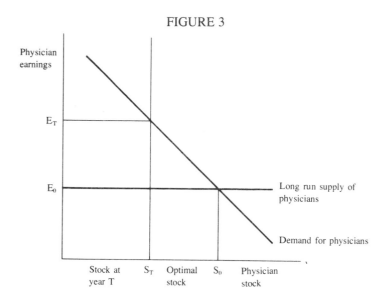

We may note also that both the moderate and the complete plan have a substantial effect on the future stocks of physicians. By the year 2000 the moderate plan has increased the stock by 71,343 or 11.6 percent over the level which would have existed with no national health plan. The complete plan results in a physician stock augmented by 216,969 in the same year. This represents a 35.4 percent increase over the anticipated number of physicians with no plan.

RESULTS WITH PRICE CONTROLS

Most advocates of NHI have recognized the potential for large, widespread fee increases. The predicted high physician fees together with the associated tax burden of financing these inflated health expenditures have therefore caused many NHI proponents to accompany their proposals with plans to limit physician fees through some form of price controls. Two general economic effects result. First, controls prevent prices from attracting resources into the production of output most valued by consumers. The restriction of price to below the market-clearing level reduces the incentive to expand supply and thus acts to prolong or even create economic shortages of the type we have been discussing. Rent controls in New York City, for example, have made it less profitable to build and maintain housing with the result that the quality and quantity of housing there have seriously deteriorated.

Price controls also cause suppliers to discriminate on the basis of factors other than price in distributing their goods and services among competing demanders. For example, a brother-in-law with a gasoline station became a highly prized relative during the 1974 gasoline "crisis." As this experience in early 1974 demonstrated, rationing according to demanders' distaste for waiting in lines is a common but wasteful way to allocate valuable resources when price is prevented from doing the job.

Both of these results are applicable to the market for physicians' services. The high earnings produced by the introduction of NHI would attract many qualified applicants enabling a rapid expansion of the future stock and thus a steady reduction of the shortage. Limiting physician fees will reduce the flow of applicants, lengthening the adjustment period.

The second effect may also be a prominent feature of the health care market with NHI. We already observe some nonprice rationing of health services. Many nonprofit clinics have chosen to give their services away "free" or to collect only nominal charges for care. One typically observes long lines (and experiences long waits) for service at such clinics. When rationing is done on the basis of waiting, however, a net social loss of resources results. This loss occurs in two forms. First, there is the waste of the waiting period itself as workers spend valuable time reading magazines in physicians' waiting rooms. Second, there is an important welfare loss as resources are discouraged by the controlled prices from going to their most valuable uses.

Our model of the physician service sector enables us to estimate the costs of price controls in this sector under the moderate or the complete national health insurance plans. We have estimated the effects of a hypothetical price control plan which calls for the government to set fees equal to the level that would have yielded equilibrium earnings in the previous year. We also assume that fee levels are readjusted every four years in the same manner.

Table 5 gives physician earnings and fees under the price control plan. The effects on the physician shortages are given in Table 6. Under the moderate health insurance plan, price controls do not produce a strong effect. Applicants to medical school were observed to respond to physician earnings with a five-year lag.[7] In turn, medical school capacity adjusts with a three-year lag to the optimal physician stock. The reduction in qualified applicants caused by price controls does not influence medical school enrollment until 1987. Since there is a minimum physician training period of five years, the stock of physicians is not affected until 1992 when supply has already fully expanded. Hence the effects of an idealized price control scheme on a moderate NHI plan is to reduce the inherent tendency to overshoot.

This is not true for the complete plan. The effect of complete NHI is assumed to be immediate. In the absence of price controls, applicants in 1982 will react to the large incomes predicted for 1977. Medical schools will also begin to adjust capacity upward by 1980. With price controls, however, medical schools would begin to be constrained by a shortage of qualified appli-

TABLE 5 Physician Earnings and Fees under Price Controls[a]

Year	Median Earnings	Median Fees
1976	44,784	9.32
1977	39,081	8.14
1978	39,081	8.14
1979	39,081	8.14
1980	39,081	8.14
1981	42,803	8.92
1982	42,803	8.92
1983	42,803	8.92
1984	42,803	8.92
1985	46,835	9.76
1986	46,835	9.76
1987	46,835	9.76
1988	46,835	9.76
1989	51,203	10.67
1990	51,203	10.67
1991	51,203	10.67
1992	51,203	10.67
1993	55,934	11.65
1994	55,934	11.65
1995	55,934	11.65
1996	55,934	11.65
1997	61,059	12.72
1998	61,059	12.72
1999	61,059	12.72
2000	61,059	12.72

[a]In 1975 dollars.

TABLE 6   The Effects of Price Controls
on the Stock of Physicians

| | Moderate NHI Plan | | Complete NHI Plan | |
| | Physician | Physician | Physician | Physician |
Year	Stock	Shortage	Stock	Shortage
1976	407,729	23,100	407,729	23,100
1977	423,061	21,595	423,061	245,760
1978	435,965	23,890	435,965	238,336
1979	448,570	28,334	453,171	226,683
1980	461,834	34,767	470,394	215,088
1981	476,290	44,151	487,638	203,546
1982	492,138	59,644	504,624	192,336
1983	509,056	48,577	521,355	181,457
1984	525,721	37,840	537,835	170,904
1985	542,136	27,428	555,568	159,175
1986	557,764	17,879	574,578	146,243
1987	570,555	11,243	592,950	134,027
1988	580,851	7,182	610,590	122,620
1989	589,612	4,731	628,082	111,440
1990	597,763	2,969	644,826	101,085
1991	605,743	1,458	662,124	90,255
1992	613,065	683	677,601	81,326
1993	619,168	1,207	691,735	73,818
1994	624,306	2,777	704,785	67,476
1995	631,365	2,506	719,637	59,412
1996	638,732	2,009	734,680	51,240
1997	646,221	1,473	749,729	43,143
1998	654,717	11	765,673	34,234
1999	663,878	−2,032	783,933	23,091
2000	673,055	−4,006	800,704	13,523

cants in 1982. Therefore by 1987 the predicted stock of physicians is reduced and the shortage increased. The adjustment period is thus lengthened and the equilibrium supply would barely be reached by the end of the century.

Table 7 shows the predicted medical school capacity under the moderate and complete insurance schemes. This table also shows the predicted number of qualified applicants under price controls and the implied medical school first-year enrollments with and without price controls. Under the moderate plan, the medical schools become constrained by the number of qualified applicants by 1987[8] and capacity would not be matched by qualified applicants again until 1995. As a result the adjustment period would increase by eight years and the number of physicians would decline 12,000 by the year 2000. For the complete plan, the effects of price controls would again be more dramatic. Once again in 1982 qualified applicants would limit medical school enrollment. Applicants would constrain enrollment until 1998. The number of physicians practicing by the year 2000 would be reduced by 30,000 relative to no price controls.

As we noted above, there are two social costs associated with the imposition of price controls. We have separately estimated (1) the costs associated with the diminished responsiveness of supply and (2) the costs imposed by a rationing system such as queuing, which itself consumes resources—i.e., forces consumers to pay part of the cost in nonmoney terms. These estimates and the techniques employed in their estimation will be discussed in turn.

Price controls, as we have seen, can have a profound effect on the applicant rate to medical school and ultimately on the supply of physicians. The social loss of this reduction in the supply of physicians is the social value placed upon their services less the social costs of producing them. In terms of Figure 4, S_T is the actual stock at a given time in the presence of price controls while S_T^* would be the stock in the absence of the controls. The social value of these additional services is approximately measured by the shaded area, E_T E_T^* S_T^* S_T. The

TABLE 7 Medical School Capacity, Qualified Applicants and First Year Enrollments, with and without Price Controls

| | Medical School Capacity | | Qualified Applicants | | | | First Year Enrollments | | | |
| | | | Moderate Plan | | Complete Plan | | Moderate Plan | | Complete Plan | |
	Moderate Plan	Complete Plan	No Price Controls	With Price Controls	No Price Controls	With Price Controls	No Price Controls	With Price Controls	No Price Controls	With Price Controls
1976	15,053	15,053	22,562	22,562	22,562	22,562	15,053	15,053	15,053	15,053
1977	15,053	15,053	20,987	20,987	20,987	20,987	15,053	15,053	15,053	15,053
1978	15,053	15,053	21,953	21,953	21,953	21,953	15,053	15,053	15,053	15,053
1979	15,053	15,053	24,061	24,061	24,061	24,061	15,053	15,053	15,053	15,053
1980	15,053	16,631	22,546	22,546	22,546	22,546	15,053	15,053	16,631	16,631
1981	15,053	18,257	22,288	22,288	22,288	22,288	15,053	15,053	18,257	18,257
1982	15,053	19,930	21,541	17,885	50,000+	17,885	15,053	15,053	19,930	17,885
1983	15,141	21,239	22,026	17,405	50,000+	17,405	15,141	15,141	21,239	17,405
1984	15,435	22,170	23,777	17,527	50,000+	17,527	15,435	15,435	22,170	17,527
1985	16,000	22,713	25,280	17,016	50,000+	17,016	16,000	16,000	22,713	17,016
1986	16,593	22,963	28,951	17,864	50,000+	17,864	16,593	16,593	22,963	17,864
1987	17,160	23,020	29,925	16,220	50,000+	16,220	17,160	16,220	23,020	16,220
1988	17,631	23,020	25,688	15,051	50,000+	15,051	17,631	15,051	23,020	15,051
1989	17,999	23,020	22,454	14,132	50,000+	14,132	17,999	14,132	23,020	14,132
1990	18,271	23,020	21,446	16,236	50,000+	16,236	18,271	16,236	23,020	16,236
1991	18,474	23,066	20,841	16,671	50,000+	16,671	18,474	16,671	23,066	16,671
1992	18,635	23,167	20,593	16,916	50,000+	16,916	18,635	16,916	23,167	16,916
1993	18,780	23,323	21,972	18,094	50,000+	18,094	18,780	18,094	23,323	18,094
1994	18,928	23,523	22,459	20,785	50,000+	20,785	18,928	18,928	23,523	20,785
1995	19,090	23,753	23,148	21,022	50,000+	21,022	19,090	19,090	23,753	21,022
1996	19,272	24,000	24,686	21,944	50,000+	21,944	19,272	19,272	24,000	21,944
1997	19,472	24,252	25,470	22,191	48,132	22,191	19,472	19,472	24,252	22,191
1998	19,689	24,502	25,591	25,188	41,209	25,188	19,689	19,689	24,502	24,502
1999	19,918	24,748	26,502	25,655	36,908	25,655	19,918	19,918	24,748	24,748
2000	20,155	24,987	25,829	24,601	31,495	24,601	20,155	20,155	24,987	24,601

FIGURE 4

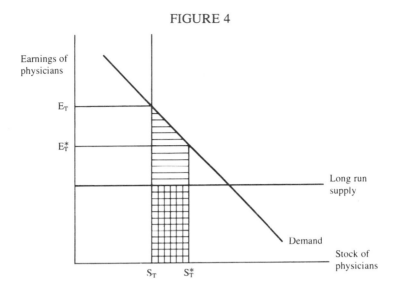

social costs of the additional stock are approximated by the area under the long-run supply curve, the crosshatched area in Figure 4. Hence, the shaded area above the long-run supply curve represents an estimate of the social costs in each time period of the price controls. Table 8 gives these losses for both the moderate and complete plans for 1976 to 2000.

Under the moderate plan, only in one year is the supply reduction a social loss, and then only of $70,000. Because of the long lags in producing physicians, the reduction in supply occurs only after adjustment has overshot the equilibrium level. Thus the principal effect of price controls on supply for the moderate plan is to mute the overshooting response. Under the complete plan the required supply adjustment is substantial. The price controls would impose a positive social cost from reducing supply as shown in Table 8. We estimate this social cost to be a maximum of $783 million in 1994. These costs, however, are quite small relative to the queuing costs.

Tables 9 and 10 report our estimates of the social loss due to queuing. Such costs are incurred if the supply of medical services is rationed by waiting in line or some other resource-using

TABLE 8   Cost of Supply Reduction Due to Price Controls[a]

Year	Moderate Plan	Complete Plan
1976	0	0
1977	0	0
1978	0	0
1979	0	0
1980	0	0
1981	0	0
1982	0	0
1983	0	0
1984	0	0
1985	0	0
1986	0	0
1987	0	114,954,800
1988	0	289,917,400
1989	0	448,931,300
1990	0	593,252,000
1991	0	653,727,400
1992	70,187	721,133,500
1993	−499,129	767,652,300
1994	−1,575,066	783,127,200
1995	−5,587,754	690,218,400
1996	−11,365,120	543,621,300
1997	−18,592,320	389,197,000
1998	−27,313,200	237,180,400
1999	−26,826,460	86,837,690
2000	−26,307,760	−9,134,912
TOTAL LOSS	−117,996,600	6,310,600,000

[a]In 1975 dollars.

method rather than by price. The explanation of this waste is quite simple, although the estimation is somewhat cumbersome. For simplicity we shall restrict our discussion to rationing by waiting, but it should be borne in mind that waiting is simply one of many resource-using methods of rationing in the absence of price.

Let us assume that the market-clearing price for the amount of services produced is $10 and the controlled price is $5. Demanders of care still value the care at $10 in spite of the controls and therefore are willing to give up $5 *plus* resources worth another $5 in order to obtain it. If the care is given away on a "first come, first serve" basis, this means that demanders will wait in line for a period up to $5-worth of time in order to purchase care at a money price of $5. As demanders all value this "low cost" care, they can be expected to join the queue and it will grow until it is long enough to discourage potential patients. They will be discouraged when waiting in line costs them $5-worth of time.[9]

Two things are clear about this process. First, in spite of controlled money price, the cost of care to potential consumers does not fall appreciably. They must still give up resources worth $10 to obtain care. It is true that the money price is less, but this decrease in the money price is *purely* cosmetic: it only forces them to pay part of the price in other forms, i.e., by waiting. The additional $5-worth of time is just as costly in terms of the consumers' welfare as $5 in money would have been.

The second fact to be noted is that resources devoted to waiting are wasted in the aggregate. The hours devoted to sitting in lines might be used in any number of productive occupations such as labor, learning, or leisure. The fact that they are consumed in obtaining care which is already produced simply raises the resource cost of this activity. The resources used to produce the care are in no way reduced by the imposition of price controls. Resources consumed in waiting add nothing to its value. They are simply lost.

TABLE 9   Cost of Rationing by Waiting Under Price Controls—Moderate Plan

Year	A.[1] Consumer Valuations When Prices Not Controlled[4]	B.[2] Consumer Valuations When Prices Are Controlled[4]	C.[3] Ratio of Controlled to Non- controlled Physician Fees	D. Implicit Consumer Price Under Price Controls[4]	E. Per Visit Cost of Rationing by Waiting[4]	F. Annual Social Cost of Rationing by Waiting[4]
1976	6.64	6.64	1.000	6.64	0.00	0
1977	6.41	6.41	0.861	5.52	0.89	3,077,709,000
1978	6.28	6.28	0.830	5.52	1.07	3,791,005,000
1979	6.17	6.17	0.791	4.88	1.29	4,720,467,000
1980	6.03	6.03	0.745	4.49	1.54	5,806,665,000
1981	5.86	5.86	0.755	4.42	1.44	5,581,512,000
1982	5.65	5.65	0.674	3.81	1.84	7,396,212,000
1983	5.42	5.42	0.703	3.81	1.61	6,676,127,000
1984	5.20	5.20	0.732	3.81	1.39	5,971,988,000
1985	5.00	5.00	0.833	4.17	0.84	3,699,354,000
1986	4.84	4.84	0.861	4.17	0.67	3,052,174,000
1987	4.76	4.76	0.876	4.17	0.59	2,750,317,000
1988	4.75	4.75	0.877	4.17	0.58	2,764,080,000
1989	4.79	4.79	0.952	4.56	0.23	1,115,698,000
1990	4.84	4.84	0.940	4.56	0.29	1,407,959,000
1991	4.91	4.91	0.928	4.56	0.35	1,745,073,000
1992	4.97	5.00	0.917	4.56	0.44	2,199,399,000
1993	5.02	5.12	0.990	4.97	0.15	747,586,500
1994	5.07	5.28	0.981	4.97	0.31	1,579,168,000
1995	5.12	5.39	0.971	4.97	0.42	2,155,549,000
1996	5.17	5.50	0.962	4.97	0.52	2,718,287,000
1997	5.22	5.60	1.040	5.43	0.17	886,878,200
1998	5.28	5.67	1.029	5.43	0.24	1,296,645,000
1999	5.34	5.73	1.018	5.43	0.30	1,616,220,000
2000	5.40	5.79	1.006	5.43	0.36	1,958,701,000

[1]Marginal valuations of physician visits implied by stocks given in Table 4 if consumers directly paid 100 percent.

[2]Marginal valuations of physician visits implied by stocks under price controls as given in Table 6 if consumers directly paid 100 percent.

[3]Ratio of fees in Table 3 and fees for price control plan, Table 5.

[4]In 1975 dollars.

TABLE 10 Cost of Rationing by Waiting Under Price Controls—Complete Plan

Year	A. Consumer Valuations When Prices Not Controlled[a]	B. Consumer Valuations When Prices Are Controlled[a]	C. Ratio of Controlled to Non-controlled Physician Fees	D. Implicit Consumer Price Under Price Controls[a]	E. Per Visit Cost of Rationing by Waiting[a]	F. Annual Social Cost of Rationing by Waiting[a]
1976	6.64	6.64	1.000	6.64	0.00	0
1977	6.41	6.41	0.231	1.48	4.93	17,018,370,000
1978	6.28	6.28	0.236	1.48	4.80	17,068,900,000
1979	6.00	6.00	0.247	1.48	4.52	16,707,200,000
1980	5.74	5.74	0.259	1.48	4.25	16,321,270,000
1981	5.48	5.48	0.297	1.63	3.86	15,347,850,000
1982	5.25	5.25	0.310	1.63	3.63	14,928,340,000
1983	5.04	5.04	0.323	1.63	3.41	14,519,400,000
1984	4.84	4.84	0.336	1.63	3.22	14,118,060,000
1985	4.62	4.62	0.385	1.78	2.85	12,898,950,000
1986	4.38	4.38	0.406	1.78	2.60	12,211,100,000
1987	4.13	4.17	0.431	1.78	2.39	11,580,250,000
1988	3.86	3.99	0.461	1.78	2.21	11,016,800,000
1989	3.61	3.82	0.539	1.95	1.88	9,613,996,000
1990	3.36	3.68	0.578	1.95	1.73	9,109,381,000
1991	3.14	3.53	0.619	1.95	1.58	8,547,983,000
1992	2.94	3.42	0.662	1.95	1.48	8,165,314,000
1993	2.76	3.35	0.770	2.12	1.22	6,906,458,000
1994	2.59	3.30	0.820	2.12	1.17	6,745,673,000
1995	2.44	3.21	0.870	2.12	1.09	6,402,764,000
1996	2.35	3.13	0.903	2.12	1.01	6,041,042,000
1997	2.31	3.05	1.002	2.32	0.73	4,486,315,000
1998	2.31	2.96	1.005	2.32	0.64	4,009,989,000
1999	2.30	2.83	1.007	2.32	0.52	3,297,902,000
2000	2.30	2.74	1.009	2.32	0.42	2,742,297,000

[a] In 1975 dollars.

The estimates in Tables 9 and 10 are obtained as follows: The resource waste per visit is estimated to be equal to the price reduction resulting from the fee ceiling. Column C in each table presents the ratio of the controlled fee to the fee that would exist in the absence of controls. Multiplying this ratio by the value which patients place on care in the absence of controls (column A in each table) gives us an implicit price which consumers would pay under price controls (column D). The implicit price reduction—and thus the resource waste per visit—is the difference in consumer valuations of care when price is controlled (column B) and the implicit price just described (column E). Multiplying this per unit loss by the predicted number of visits in each year gives the annual social waste resulting from rationing by waiting. This is shown in column F.[10]

As expected, the loss due to rationing far exceeds that of the supply reduction. The potential loss under the moderate plan reaches over $7 billion in 1982 when price controls would most constrain the market. Throughout the estimated period the cost to the economy would average nearly $3 billion. This represents a pure loss to the economy whether occurring through increased absence from work or reduced leisure. The effects under the complete plan are, of course, even more dramatic. The price controls act to reduce price to less than one-fourth its market-clearing value in the initial periods. The large increase in demand would produce very large queues and true tests of consumer stamina. The potential costs to the economy in the first year alone will be over $17 billion. The social costs would potentially average nearly $10 billion a year over the twenty-five year period until 2000.

Though these estimates are preliminary, we believe them to be indicative of the potential damage which price controls may cause. These costs certainly can be avoided by making entitlement to medical care arbitrary, i.e., not under the control of those desiring care. By assigning appointments on the basis of random drawings, for example, an NHI system might avoid the incentive to devote resources to wasteful activities like waiting in line. Unfortunately, elimination of waste via this method introduces waste of another. Random assignments of appointments would, of course, fail in any sense to apportion appointments to those individuals to whom they are most valuable. Proponents of controls—those wishing to eliminate economic considerations from such allocative decisions as who will be treated by physicians—would ideally like to have these resources allocated by physicians. That is, they would like a strictly medical determination of need to govern who obtains the scarce care available.[11] There is little in this ideal with which economists can take exception. Unfortunately, such a scheme is simply not feasible organizationally. A physician really would have to see such individuals in order to screen out the undeserving from those whose conditions truly warrant attention. Yet it is precisely this sort of attention (weighing of reported systems and deciding on the need for treatment) which occupies most physician time under the present regime. Providing all the demanders who would appear for zero-priced medical attention with one such screening visit would more than exhaust the time of all physicians now providing patient care. No time would remain to make treatment available to those deemed worthy.

A more realistic alternative widely employed by the English National Health Service is to ration the limited care produced on the basis of time preference. For nonemergency items such as elective surgery, names are simply added to a queue which may extend several years into the future. Those willing to wait the required time eventually receive the care prescribed. Those unwilling to wait purchase the care they desire from the limited private sector which exists essentially to serve this market. Unfortunately, with all-pervasive price controls as a part of national health insurance in this country, a secondary market such as this could not exist and rationing on the basis of time preference is not feasible either. Having no alternative, those desiring care would all remain on the list and as long as demand continues to exceed supply such a list would simply get longer and longer over time. It would, in short, not operate as a rationing device.

Ultimately, then, given controls on physician fees, it seems to us that it will be impossible to avoid using some resource-consuming form of rationing. It may be found that some of these costs may be reduced or eliminated for certain types of care. We must nevertheless urge that such a combination of programs be given the gravest sort of consideration. The system potentially could waste as much as $17 billion per year. The government and the private sector combined are currently spending only $22 billion on physician services, so such a loss must be deemed substantial.

SUMMARY

In this chapter we have provided estimates of the effects on the price and quantity supplied of physician services under two alternative national health insurance proposals: a moderate program phased in over a five-year period which eventually covers up to 90 percent of all medical care expenditures, and a complete plan adopted immediately which covers all medical care expenditures. The price effects of both plans are predicted to be substantial. Fees rise under the moderate plan by as much as 42 percent while under the complete plan they rise by as much as 277 percent. These inflationary effects are fully dissipated for the moderate plan by the year 1990 but prevail virtually to the end of the century for the complete plan. Quantity effects are also substantial. The moderate plan would increase the quantity of physicians by 12 percent by 1990 while the complete plan would result in a 23 percent increase in the number of physicians.

This chapter also estimates the effect on this market of imposing controls over fees. Depending on the insurance plan, fee ceilings were predicted to have differing effects on the adjustment process. For the moderate plan the cost were trivial, as the delay imposed on the adjustment process was found to just offset the current overshooting effect resulting from the imposition of Medicare and Medicaid. Delays in the adjustment to the complete plan were of another order of magnitude. Full adjustment is not predicted before the end of the century for a system of complete coverage of the type modeled here combined (almost certainly) with price controls. Costs imposed by these delays would be negligible compared to those associated with non–price rationing. Waiting costs were predicted to be as much as $17 billion in this category.

APPENDIX
THE EQUATIONS USED TO MODEL THE
MARKET FOR PHYSICIAN SERVICES

1. Earnings equation[12]

$$\text{Log}(E_T) = -.000005862 \cdot S_T + .72922 \cdot \text{Log}(Y_T) +$$
$$(-6.812) \qquad (2.28)$$
$$.0016692\ P_T - .3696\ \text{Log}(D_T) + 1.9415$$
$$(6.912) \qquad (-2.655) \qquad (1.833)$$

$$R^2 = .9848,\ DW = 1.488$$

where E_T is net general practitioner median earnings before
taxation, year T;
S_T is the stock of physicians in private practice in year T;
Y_T is real family income in year T;
P_T is the population in thousands in year T;
D_T is the percentage of expenditures on physician services
paid directly by consumers.

2. Profitability equation

$$\Pi_t = \sum_{i=1}^{58} \left(\frac{EP_{iT} - OC_{iT}}{(1 + .1)^i} \right)$$

where Π_T is the pecuniary return to physician training
estimated in year T;

EP_{iT} is median physician earnings at age $21+i$, in
year T, adjusted for expected mortality, taxation, differential work hours and military
service. This variable includes all schooling
costs;

OC_{iT} is the opportunity costs, assumed to be those of
the median college graduate, at age $21+i$ in
year T adjusted as above. [13]

3. Applicant equation

$$Log (A_T) = .0000155908 \cdot \Pi_{T-5} + .00124182 \cdot CG_T$$
$$(2.761) \qquad\qquad (7.145)$$
$$+9.09938$$
$$(9.965) \qquad\qquad R^2 = .9767, DW = 1.4$$

where A_T is the number of applicants to medical school in
year T;

Π_T is profitability as defined in 2;

CG_T is the number of college graduates in year T.

4. Optimal medical school capacity

$$OCAP_T = .033 \cdot OS_T - 1000$$

where $OCAP_T$ is the optimal medical school capacity in year T;

OS_T is the optimal stock of physicians in year T defined
as that stock which yields an earnings level via 1
that in turn yields a zero profitability via 2.

The coefficient on OS_T is estimated from mortality tables
and retirement at age 70 such that $.033 \cdot OS_T$ will be expected to leave practice annually in steady state equilibrium.
One thousand is substracted as expected foreign-trained
physician inflow in equilibrium.

5. Medical school capacity

$$CAP_T = .26222 \cdot (OCAP_{T-3} - CAP_{T-3}) + CAP_{T-1}$$
$$(4.76) \qquad\qquad\qquad R^2 = .5478$$

where CAP_T is the medical school capacity in year T;
   $OCAP_T$ is the optimal capacity in year T as defined in 4.

The adjustment coefficient was estimated in a separate regression of the change in capacity regressed on various lags of optimal capacity shortage.

6. Newly licensed American physicians

$$G_T = .95 \cdot MIN(CAP_{T-5}, .5 \cdot A_{T-5})$$

where G_T is newly licensed American trained physicians;
   CAP_T is medical school capacity as in 5;
   A_T is applicants as in 3.

This equation assumes 5 percent medical school noncompletion and a first year enrollment constraint of either capacity in year T or one-half applicants in year T, whichever is less.

7. Foreign-trained physician inflow

$$F_T = 1000, \text{ if } .25 \cdot SHPS_{T-2} < 1000$$
$$F_T = .25 \cdot SHPS_{T-2} \text{ if } 1000 < .25 \cdot SHPS_{T-2} < 10,000$$
$$F_T = 10,000, \text{ if } .25 \cdot SHPS_{T-2} > 10,000$$

where F_T is foreigners licensed in year T;
   $SHPS_T$ is the physician shortage in year T, defined as the optimal stock, OPS_T in 4, minus the actual stock S_T in 1.

This equation assumes foreign physicians will make up one-quarter of the shortage lagged two years back, with a minimum inflow of one thousand and a maximum inflow of ten thousand.

8. The physician stock

$$S_T = .985 \cdot S_{T-1} + F_T + G_T$$

All as defined above.

9. Future population, future family income, future college graduates, and future opportunity costs, 1975–2000.

Population is assumed to grow at an annual rate of 1 percent. Family income is assumed to grow at a rate of 2.5 percent. Median college graduate's income is assumed to grow at a rate of 2 percent. Future college graduates are from estimates in *Projections of Educational Statistics,* U.S. Office of Education, and interpolation.

The coefficients on equations 1, 3, and 5 were estimated using ordinary least squares on data from 1947 to 1973. The expected dropout rate in equation 6 is the historical average for medical schools. The expected retirement rate in equation 8, i.e., the coefficient on S_{T-1}, is estimated from mortality tables for a stock growing at a constant rate of 2 percent. All data utilized in estimations is found in Leffler, "Licensure in Medicine" (Ph.D. dissertation, University of California, Los Angeles, in progress).

10

ALAIN ENTHOVEN

Does Anyone Want Competition? The Politics of NHI

Tax exclusions and the development of health insurance. Fair competition in health care plans. The Consumer-Choice Health Plan. Congressional studies. Labor, business, the medical profession, hospitals, and the commercial health insurance industry. Blue Cross/Blue Shield in a competitive system.

TODAY'S LACK OF COMPETITION

Health services in the United States today are, for the most part, not organized on the basis of *economic competition* in the usual sense of that term. In normal economic competition, buyers and sellers are cost conscious. Buyers have limited budgets. If they spend more for one good, they have less to spend on others. Producers of goods and services face market prices and they pay the full cost of the resources they use in production. If they spend more on some resource, their net incomes are reduced. Competition in such a framework rewards both buyers and sellers for economy in the use of resources.

These are not the rules that govern our health services economy. Most consumers have insurance which pays all or the largest part of their medical bills, so consumers have little or no economic incentive to question the need for the health services they receive or the value of them. Most health insurance offers a "free choice of doctor," effectively ruling out economic competition among doctors. That is, the patient's insurance premium will be virtually the same whether he chooses the most extravagant or the most economical doctor. Most insurance pays doctors on fee-for-service or piecework bases, which means that the doctor is paid more for providing more services whether or not more produce any benefit for the patient. Moreover, doctors generally are paid more per unit of their time for providing high technology care in high cost settings.

Hospitals are paid either on the basis of costs or charges. Medicare, Medicaid, and many Blue Cross plans pay on the basis of cost reimbursement which rewards hospitals for generating more costs. The real buyers of hospital services are usually not price conscious. The doctors who order the services have little reason to care about charges. Their patients, for the most part, are insured for the cost of hospital services. Insurers may object that some charges are "unreasonable" but "reasonableness" is judged mainly in relation to cost.

Health insurers compete with each other and with employer self-funded health insurance, but this competition is only over the amount of the insurer's administrative costs and profit margins, which typically are only roughly 10 percent of total premium costs. For the most part, ability to control the costs of health *services* is not a factor in this competition. The power to control costs is the power not to buy if the price isn't right, but insurers don't have this power. Patients and doctors make the buying decisions. In a world of "free choice of doctor" insurance, economic competition in health insurance is not effectively translated into economic competition in health services.

MEDICARE AND MEDICAID

The great majority of Americans are insured either through Medicare if they are aged or disabled, through Medicaid if they are poor and fit a category that is covered, or through an employer-provided health insurance plan. Medicare is a federal program, financed largely by payroll taxes with some general revenues. It pays for covered hospital services on the basis of cost reimbursement and for covered physician services on the basis of fee-for-service. After an annual deductible of $60, Medicare pays 80 percent of physicians' fees for covered services up to 80 percent of "reasonable charges." Actual charges often substantially exceed what the Health Care Financing Administration considers to be reasonable. In such cases, the patient pays the difference and can benefit from choosing a doctor whose fees are lower. But physician gross incomes are only about 16 percent of total health care costs (not including laboratory tests billed through their offices), while hospital costs are about 40 percent of the total. For hospitalization, after a deductible for each "spell of illness" (equal to $144 in 1978), Medicare pays all the cost of covered services for the first sixty days. This covers the great majority of hospitalizations. So the patient realizes little or no economic benefit from choosing doctors who use hospitalization economically.

As a result, Medicare pays more on behalf of patients who choose doctors who perform more services and order more hospital services for a given medical condition. For example, a study of Medicare experience with six prepaid group practice plans revealed that, on average, Medicare paid 36 percent more on behalf of beneficiaries who were cared for under insured fee-for-service than on behalf of patients matched by age, sex, and location, and therefore presumably of equal medical need, cared for by the less-costly prepaid group practices. In one case Medicare paid 76 percent more on behalf of the beneficiaries who chose fee-for-service. Medicare thus acts as a major barrier to fair economic competition between fee-for-service doctors and prepaid group practice doctors.

Similarly, Medicaid pays providers of care on the basis of cost reimbursement and fee-for-service. While the allowable fees and costs may be less than what the providers of care consider customary or their true costs, no charge to the patient is allowed. Generally speaking, then, there is no reward to the Medicaid patient for seeking out more economical providers. Medicaid too acts as a barrier to fair economic competition among providers.

THE TAX LAWS AND EMPLOYER HEALTH PLANS

Employer contributions to employee health benefits are excluded from the employees' taxable income, an exclusion estimated to cost the federal and state governments about $14 billion in foregone revenues in 1979. This particular form of tax preference has had profound consequences on the development of health insurance in this country and has been an important influence in creating another major barrier to economic competition in health services.

The tax exclusion has put the control of health benefits under employers or, where there are unions, jointly under the control of labor and management. But labor and management have their own purposes, and using this control to create a competitive market for health care services in their communities has not been one of them. Rather, health benefits have been seen largely as a prize to be won or yielded at the bargaining table, or as a tool to be used to attract qualified employees to the firm and to retain them. Thus the predominant pattern is a single employer-provided health benefits plan offering the employee "free choice of doctor."

Furthermore, the incentive inherent in the tax laws motivates employers and employees to agree that it is in their mutual interest for the employer to pay 100 percent of whatever health benefits the employees want to buy. Employees can get much more with their employer's pre-tax dollars than with their own net-after-tax dollars. Thus the tax exclusion has encouraged 100 percent employer-paid comprehensive benefits including first-dollar coverage. While there may be a substantial cost in economic efficiency attributable to making services free to employees, this is apparently offset from the employee group's point of view by the tax advantage.

Finally, the tax exclusion means more tax-free compensation for employees who choose more costly health plans.

How this works to block competition in health services can be illustrated by an example. In San Mateo County, California, many employees were offered a choice in 1978 between a comprehensive insured fee-for-service plan and membership in the Kaiser-Permanente prepaid group practice plan. The typical family premium for the former was roughly $125 per month, depending on the particular group. The typical family premium for the latter was about $85 per month. *Many employers paid 100 percent of the premium either way*, and in so doing sent an unmistakable signal to the more costly providers that there was no need for them to compete on an economic basis.

Two new individual practice associations were seeking to enter the market in San Mateo County, each offering comprehensive services for about $110 per family per month. Their market entry was retarded by the fact that many employees could get care from the same providers either through an insured fee-for-service plan or through the individual practice association. While the employee made the choice among plans, the employer paid the premium. (To get care from Kaiser doctors, the employee had to join the Kaiser plan.) Thus the employee who made the decision got no financial reward for making an economical choice. To the extent this pattern predominated, there was no market for cost control and no possibility of competition.

A survey of employer health plan offerings in Santa Clara County in 1979 revealed that, of employers with five hundred or more employees, 36 percent offered their employees a single health insurance plan, 42 percent offered a choice but contributed more on behalf of the employee choosing the more costly alternative, and only 22 percent offered a choice and an equal employer contribution. Of employers with between twenty-five and five hundred employees, 73 percent offered employees no choice, 23 percent offered a choice but paid more on behalf of the employees choosing the more costly plan, and only 3 percent offered both a choice and an equal contribution. Of those offering a choice, one-third of the larger employers and three-quarters of the smaller employers paid 100 percent of the premium, whichever plan the employee chose. Because of the size and longevity of the Kaiser program there, one would expect employers in Santa Clara County to be much more likely than most employers to offer choices and encourage competition.

As these data suggest, we are very far from a fair economic competition in health services, even in California.

PRINCIPLES OF COMPETITION

A system of fair economic competition among health care financing and delivery plans would be based on the following principles.

Periodic multiple choice.   Each consumer would be offered, periodically, the opportunity to enroll in any one of the health plans operating in his or her area and meeting certain uniform standards governing all health plans.

Fixed dollar subsidies. The amount of financial help each consumer would get toward the purchase of a health plan membership—from Medicare, Medicaid, an employer, or through the tax laws—would be in the form of a fixed dollar amount that was the same regardless of the plan he or she chose. (The subsidy might vary by geography, income, or demographic category.) Thus, consumers who chose more costly health plans would pay the extra cost themselves; consumers who chose less costly plans would save money. Buyers in this market would thus be cost conscious.

Equal rules for all competitors. A workable system of health plan competition must be based on a uniform set of rules to assure that all health plans are competing to provide good quality comprehensive care at a reasonable cost and are not profiting by such practices as selection of preferred risks or selling deceptive or inadequate coverage. Rules would have to be established governing enrollment procedures, premium-setting practices, minimum standards for covered benefits, and information disclosure.

Organization of doctors into competing economic units. There would be no economic competition in health services if the other principles were applied but if all doctors participated equally in the health care plans. Rather, some "limited provider plans" (sometimes called "closed panel plans") would have to be established. Patients selecting such plans accept a limited choice of doctor, including only those participating in or contracting with that particular plan, in exchange for what they perceive to be better benefits or lower costs. Premiums then reflect the cost-generating experience of the doctors in each plan. Economical doctors can attract more patients by offering a lower premium. While traditional insurance plans offering "free choice of doctor" would be included among the choices and some doctors would continue to practice on a fee-for-service basis, competition would almost certainly encourage the development of "alternative delivery systems"—the limited provider plans such as prepaid group practices, individual practice associations, and primary care networks, all with built-in cost controls.

For the most part, these principles of competition are not applied in the U.S. health services economy today. They are, however, applied in a few places with considerable success— most notably in Minneapolis—St. Paul and Hawaii. Based on these experiences, it seems reasonable to project that thorough-going application of competitive principles would transform the health services economy, gradually and voluntarily, from today's system with cost-increasing incentives to one with built-in cost controls and incentives for consumer satisfaction.

A good example of the large-scale application of these principles is the Federal Employees Health Benefits Program (FEHBP), in successful operation since 1960 and now covering about ten million people. The government makes a fixed monthly contribution per individual or family. The worker is offered a multiple choice of private health plans and pays the difference, through payroll deduction, between the premium on the plan of his or her choice and the government contribution. More than eighty private health plans participate. The system is remarkable for its simplicity and ease of administration.

CONSUMER-CHOICE HEALTH PLAN

In the spring of 1977 President Carter reaffirmed his support for a universal and comprehensive system of national health insurance. That summer, as a special consultant to HEW Secretary Joseph Califano, I designed a proposal called Consumer-Choice Health Plan (CCHP) based on fair economic competition of alternative health care financing and delivery plans.

Briefly, the plan would replace today's tax subsidies for the non-aged, non-poor with a refundable tax credit usable only as a premium contribution toward a qualified health care financing and delivery plan. A qualified health plan would be one obeying certain rules outlined below. In the full version of CCHP, the tax credit would equal 60 percent of the actuarial cost for covered services for people in each demographic category. The present Medicare system would be replaced by a system of premium subsidies in fixed dollar amounts equal in real value to the average cost to Medicare today of people in each demographic category. In addition to the tax credits, Medicaid would be replaced by a system of premium subsidies which would be on a sliding scale, inversely related to income, and equal to 100 percent of actuarial cost in the case of the very poor. Competing private health plans would quote premiums by demographic category. People in higher medical risk categories would pay higher premiums (so that health plans would be adequately compensated for serving them) and receive correspondingly higher subsidies.

To be eligible to receive these tax-credit and other subsidy revenues, a qualified health plan would have to comply with the following rules. First, it would have to participate in an annual *open enrollment* in which it would have to accept all enrollees who chose it without regard to age, sex, race, religion, national origin, or prior medical conditions. The government would manage the process in a manner analogous to that used in the successful Federal Employees Health Benefits Program in such a way as to assure that everybody was given a full and free choice. Second, each plan would practice *community rating*, charging the same premium to all persons in the same demographic category enrolled for the same benefits in the same geographic area. Third, all plans would have to insure a common set of legally defined basic health services. They would have to offer one option limited to such services. They would also have to provide "catastrophic expense protection," limiting each family's annual out-of-pocket expenses for basic health services.

Finally, they would have to participate in a program of information disclosure designed to facilitate informed consumer choice.

Consumer-Choice Health Plan was not adopted by the Carter administration. While it attracted considerable support by economists in the administration, most of the key people associated with HEW opposed it. The latter were already fully committed to a regulatory approach to cost control, as exemplified by the administration's twice-defeated Hospital Cost Containment proposal.

INCREMENTAL PROPOSALS
FOR REFORM

One response to CCHP was congressional and Domestic Policy Council inquiries about the possibility of low-cost incremental proposals designed to foster both economic competition in health services and the growth of alternative delivery systems without instituting a full universal health insurance scheme. In February 1979 I presented the following proposals for incremental reform.

First, as a condition for continued favorable tax treatment of employer-provided health benefits, every employer above a certain size should be required to offer his employees a choice of at least three distinct health care financing and delivery plans meeting certain standards. (Three "options" from the same carrier would not meet the requirement.) Second, the employer's contribution should have to be the same whichever plan the employee chooses. Third, all qualifying plans would have to include coverage of standard basic minimum benefits, "catastrophic expense protection," and continuity of coverage provisions.

I also recommended a proposal previously developed by leaders of the Health Maintenance Organization (HMO) industry and subsequently sponsored by the Carter administration that would permit each Medicare beneficiary to direct that his average cost to the Medicare program (calculated as the "adjusted average per capita cost" for people in his actuarial category who are not members of an HMO) be paid, as a premium contribution on his behalf, to the HMO of his choice in the form of a fixed prospective payment. This would require Medicare to contribute equally on behalf of people choosing fee-for-service and HMOs. (Actually, the Carter administration proposal was for a premium contribution to HMOs equal to 95 percent of equality to permit the government to share in any savings.) Ways and Means Committee Chairman Al Ullman, Senator David Durenberger, and other key congressional leaders have endorsed these proposals and introduced legislation to put them into effect.

The direction of the health care economy is set by the balance of many complex forces. Proposals to create competition thus must be designed with some care. Not all forms of competition would be viable or desirable. For example, some have proposed that employees be given an annual choice between a comprehensive health insurance plan, such as one offered by an HMO, and an insurance plan whose premium is kept very low by use of high coinsurance and deductibles, with the employees who choose the low-cost plan being allowed to receive the difference in premiums in the form of tax-free cash rebates. The trouble with such a competition is that it could not be fair with respect to the risks insured. People expecting low medical costs would choose the low-cost plan. When they expected substantial medical expenses, they would switch to the comprehensive plan until their medical needs were taken care of, then switch back. (A great deal of the need for medical care is predictable or controllable with respect to timing.) The comprehensive plans could not survive such a competition. The resulting situation would be unlikely to produce effective cost control or affordable insurance for persons with high medical risks.

WHO WANTS COMPETITION?

The principal interest groups have reacted in diverse ways to these proposals. None of them aggressively supports competition over the status quo. But the leaders of some groups perceive that the status quo is untenable. The rapid increase in costs is forcing the government to act to get costs under control. We have been drifting into direct government controls on prices, capacity, and use of services. Some of the key groups perceive that to be less desirable than competition. There is thus reason to hope that a system of fair economic competition might be a compromise acceptable to most groups.

Organized Labor

The labor movement has a long-standing commitment to universal social insurance, including a single comprehensive standard of health care for everyone as a matter of right. In the labor view, services should be provided on the basis of medical need, and neither the cost of care nor the ability to pay should be a factor in the patient's use of services. Union leaders do not share the economists' view of the market as an efficient or appropriate allocator of resources. They share instead the traditional "liberal" (in the American sense of the term) faith in government as the instrument of desirable social change.

The principles of the Consumer Choice Health Plan are not incompatible with universal health insurance at a high—if not single—standard of comprehensive care. But CCHP's emphasis on diversity and choice appears to labor leaders to conflict with their emphasis on raising a single standard of care. As a matter of priority, they believe getting everyone covered by comprehensive health insurance is more important than getting each person covered by the system and style of care he prefers. At best, if CCHP is not incompatible with universal health insurance at an acceptable standard of care, it is seen as a diversion from the main struggle. Labor has not considered it a welcome or useful attempt to achieve universal health insurance in a way acceptable to most Americans.

Moreover, the rhetoric of competition and incentives for efficiency is unpalatable to the labor point of view. As one economist explained to me, "what sounds like efficient allocation to you sounds like a speed-up to them." So far, labor leaders have not appreciated the fact that the purpose of the proposals is to make *doctors* compete to *serve workers.* The idea that it is possible to take some aspects of resource allocation out of the market (for example, not allowing insurers to practice preferred-risk selection) while leaving other aspects in the market is a fairly subtle and recent idea and not likely to be very appealing to someone who mistrusts markets to begin with.

In collective bargaining, the traditional goal of labor has been to have the employer pay 100 percent of comprehensive health benefits. Here social philosophy has been reinforced by the tax laws which make such benefits tax-free to the employee. On the way to this goal, health benefits have provided labor leaders an apparently inexhaustible source of bargaining prizes with names that have emotional appeal. It has thus been very important for labor leaders to be able to bargain for and control entitlements to employer-paid health services. Also, solidarity in the bargaining process depends on everyone being treated alike. Lots of individual options can diffuse the force of a bargaining position.

These ideas conflict with the notion that each employer should offer a fixed-dollar contribution toward the health plan of the worker's choice and that each worker should be offered a multiple choice of health plans. Labor leaders feel that such proposals interfere with labor/management negotiations, take away authority from the unions and give it to individual workers. As one labor leader explained: "We like one health plan. We can handle two. But a choice of six is too much every man for himself."

Both CCHP and the bills introduced by Congressman Ullman and Senator Durenberger include changes in the tax laws that would limit tax-free employer contributions to health insurance. But some unions are among the groups that receive the largest employer contributions. For example, in 1979 Chrysler was paying over $2,800 per year on behalf of auto workers with families getting their care through Michigan Blue Cross/Blue Shield. Such groups would be almost bound to lose from a change in the tax laws that gave an equal tax subsidy to all families.

Labor leaders like prepaid group practice and dislike fee-for-service, which confronts them with a dilemma. Traditionally they have fought for comprehensive benefits as opposed to limited benefits with high coinsurance and deductibles. This has been favorable to prepaid group practices which traditionally offer comprehensive benefits. It is difficult for prepaid group practices to compete against limited insurance plans with high deductibles and coinsurance because, where consumers have such a choice, those expecting few medical expenses will take the low-premium insurance and leave the prepaid group to suffer from adverse risk selection. In recent years, however, the benefits covered by negotiated insured fee-for-service plans have become quite comprehensive, and the premiums often exceed the premiums for prepaid group practice plans. In 1979, for example, the Michigan Blue Cross/Blue Shield monthly premium for a Chrysler auto worker and family was about $207; the Health Alliance prepaid group premium was $143. The practice of requiring the employer to pay 100 percent of the premium has come to mean forcing employers to subsidize fee-for-service against prepaid group practice.

Somehow labor leaders will have to modify their position to resolve the dilemma. One interim step would be to negotiate for an employer contribution for all workers equal to 100 percent of the cost of the insured fee-for-service plan while allowing workers choosing less costly prepaid group practice to apply the savings to other benefits. Indeed, such arrangements—described in the Revenue Act of 1978 as "Cafeteria Style Benefit Plans"— already exist. While this approach conflicts with the idea of uniform benefits for all, it can reconcile 100 percent employer payment and fair economic competition. The difficulty is that such a solution leaves the employer contribution tied to the costs of fee-for-service which are rising too fast. Some other standard is needed. Labor now supports the new Kennedy plan, the Health Care for All Americans Act. In that proposal, health plans that can deliver comprehensive benefits for a community-rated premium less than the government-mandated ceiling would be allowed to make cash rebates to their enrollees as a way of attracting their business. In fact, the new Kennedy plan does allow for limited competition in the private sector. Some have described it as an attempt to reconcile the previous proposal, Health Security, with the principles of competition.

Business

There has been no comparable, unified view among business leaders. Businessmen understand the principles of competition and generally approve of them as long as they are not applied to their own industry. Perhaps the most realistic measure of their views about competition in health services is their actual behavior as employers. Some employers have taken a positive view toward health plan competition. In the early 1970s, for example, a group of employers in Minneapolis—St. Paul studied the problem of health care costs and decided to encourage competition. In 1970 there was one Health Maintenance Organization in the area with 36,000 members. By 1979 there were seven, with a combined membership exceeding 300,000. The support and encouragement of employers was a decisive factor in that development.

Leading employers in Minneapolis—St. Paul offer their employees a multiple choice of health plans. Control Data, for example, offers a choice of five plans; Honeywell offers six. Leading employers located elsewhere have also embraced the concept of health plan competition. Hewlett-Packard and IBM have adopted the policy of offering their employees the opportunity to join any federally qualified HMO serving their area. However, recall that only a minority of employers offer their employees a choice of health plans on an economically fair basis. So, for the most part, employers have not applied competitive principles to their own purchases of health care services.

Several factors appear to contribute to the dominant employer practice of not offering choices. First, most still think of traditional insured fee-for-service as the normal and appropriate way to buy health care services. They think of alternative delivery systems such as prepaid group practice, individual practice associations, and primary care networks as something suspect, possibly second rate, or only applicable to Californians. Indeed, the idea of health plan choices only makes much sense in the context of alternative delivery systems. But alternative delivery systems haven't existed in most areas until recently. There is a "chicken and egg" problem: the alternatives can't get started because the employers don't offer fair choices, and employers don't offer choices because the alternatives don't exist.

Employee benefit managers often react to the idea of offering choices with concern that it means more administrative work for them or would upset existing insurance arrangements.

Many employers take a short-run and company-specific view. They think in terms of health benefits as a tool to be used for attracting and retaining employees. Thus they want to be able to say they offer a "better" health plan, not merely an opportunity to buy membership in the same health plans offered by other employers. Some find health benefits to be valuable bargaining pawns in the collective bargaining process.

Other employers focus on the premium cost alone, and not on the total of premium and out-of-pocket costs. Health Maintenance Organizations often have higher premium costs because their premiums cover comprehensive services. They also frequently have lower total costs. Employers who look only at premiums often conclude, incorrectly, that "HMOs cost more."

There is some benefit to the individual employer from offering choices. The employees get more value from the employer's dollar if they are given distinctive alternatives. But the main benefits of competition come with the lower rate of growth of health care costs when most employees in an area are offered a fair choice. Although health care costs may now be a large item, a company must perceive that it can gain a competitive advantage over other companies before it will be motivated to invest resources in health care cost reduction. Yet economic competition is likely to benefit all employers in a community. The incentive to be the first ones to lead the way is not strong.

Employer resistance to offering choices is gradually breaking down, but it is a slow process.

At the level of national legislation, it is still too soon to tell how business will respond to pro-competitive legislation. Some business leaders have already endorsed an approach to health care cost control based on incentives and competition in the private sector. The National Chamber of Commerce has supported this approach. Other business organizations and leaders are likely to do so. However, the force of their support will be attenuated by other legislative priorities.

Medical Profession

The medical profession traditionally has opposed economic competition in health care services. For example, it has insisted on the principle that every insurance plan should provide for "free choice of doctor." This principle is opposed to the principle that every consumer should have the right to limit his choice of doctor, voluntarily, in exchange for what he perceives to be better benefits or lower costs. The medical profession has resisted attempts by insurance plans to discriminate between participating providers who accept cost controls and nonparticipating providers who do not, and it has backed its resistance with boycotts of "limited provider" insurance plans. The profession has ostracized and otherwise retaliated against doctors participating in prepaid group practices.

Today the profession faces a dilemma. The noncompetitive insured fee-for-service system is clearly associated with the rapidly increasing cost of health care services. And this cost increase is causing a serious financial problem for government. Public sector spending on health services increased from $11 billion in 1965 to $78 billion in 1978. Government is being forced to act to get this spending under control. Up to now, its principal response has been public utility–type bureaucratic controls on prices and utilization which most doctors like even less than the prospects of economic competition. Moreover, circumstances are gradually forcing them to make a choice. The *status quo* is becoming untenable.

In October 1976 the Board of Trustees of the American Medical Association established an independent National Commission on the Cost of Medical Care with a distinguished membership representative of business, health insurers, hospitals, independent scholars, and legislators, as well as physicians associated with the AMA. The commission faced the dilemma of competition versus regulation, and in December 1977 came down on the side of competition. Their recommendations included economic incentives in purchasing insurance and health plans (offering employees choices, employer contributions that are equal with respect to the health plan chosen, equal tax treatment), consumer cost sharing, fair market health plan competition, and alternative financing arrangements. In June 1978 the AMA House of Delegates gave a cautious and limited endorsement to the recommendations of the national commission. Other physicians also have favored economic competition. In September 1978 the American Association of Foundations for Medical Care—the association of physicians involved in Individual Practice Associations—endorsed CCHP.

There appears to be a great deal of ambivalence about competition in the leadership of the AMA and among physicians in general. Some of this ambivalence may reflect the fact that the short-term economic interest of the medical profession is in maintaining the *status quo*. The AMA's 1979 lobbying efforts focused on defeating the Carter administration's proposed Hospital Cost Containment bill and not on formulating and backing proposals to enhance competition. In the circumstances, AMA leaders could not oppose competition, since many of their allies in the fight against cost containment favored competition as a means of controlling cost. So AMA leaders have endorsed competition in a very general way that leaves them ample room to oppose specific pro-competitive steps. For example, in 1979 they opposed an administration proposal for (almost) a fair HMO option for Medicare beneficiaries whereby Medicare would pay 95 percent of the fee-for-service average cost (actuarially adjusted) on behalf of beneficiaries who choose to enroll in an HMO. To some, AMA leaders left the distinct impression that they considered economic competition in health services to be unworkable.

Hospitals

The *status quo* also has important advantages for hospitals. They now face a growing demand that is not price sensitive. Cost reimbursement relieves their managements of the burden of hard economic choices. But this situation also has important disadvantages for them. Because hospital spending is the largest and one of the fastest growing components of total health care spending, government cost containment efforts have naturally focused on it. So hospital administrators have found themselves entangled in an increasingly complex web of regulation. Costs under Medicare are reimbursed, but subject to a complex set of limits and disallowances so that reimbursements fall short of actual costs. A constant struggle by both hospitals and government to bend accounting rules to their respective benefit has produced a situation of unbelievable complexity. New investments cannot be made without certificates-of-need, and this process has proved to be very expensive, time consuming, and highly political.

In the past, some hospital industry leaders have favored state rate regulation in the belief that they could be the dominant influence on the regulatory agencies. They saw regulatory agencies as setting rates that would cover their costs and protect them from attempts by some third-party payors to pay less than full cost. However, industry leaders saw the Carter administration's Hospital Cost Containment proposal as likely to subject hospitals to permanent detailed and often perverse federal controls. Caught between the growing demand fueled by insured fee-for-service and the government's cost control efforts, the hospitals find themselves in an increasingly uncomfortable position.

Hospital industry leaders know that prepaid group practices and some other types of HMO typically hospitalize their patients 25 to 45 percent less than similar people cared for under insured fee-for-service. This is the main way such organizations hold down costs. So economic competition among such organized systems is likely to reduce considerably the demand for hospital services. However, industry leaders also know that hospitals will always be needed, that some demand for inpatient services would be replaced by demand for hospital outpatient services, and that hospitals would be able to adapt to competition in many ways, including that of converting space from acute care use to long-term care or ambulatory care facilities. Generally speaking, hospital administrators look forward to a leading role in a more organized health care delivery system.

While none of the national hospital associations has yet taken a formal position on proposed legislation, the leadership of these associations has been generally quite positive towards competition. This might be a stratagem for defeating the Carter administration's Hospital Cost Containment proposal, but support for competition appears to run deeper. Hospital industry leaders recognize that the government will be forced to do something very fundamental about controlling costs. They generally take the long view and acknowledge their choice to be between detailed federal controls and a system of true economic competition. In the latter situation, hospital administrators would be facing local private sector buyers, such as health maintenance organizations, who are conscious of quality as well as cost, informed about local conditions, and empowered to make decisions based on judgment—all quite the opposite from what they would face in federal price control authorities. Under competition, they would be rewarded for finding ways to provide better care at less cost. For these reasons hospital administrators give considerable support to competition.

Commercial Health Insurance Industry

The commercial health insurance industry opposes proposals to create competition in health services such as CCHP and the incremental proposals described above. Since open opposition would put the industry in an embarrassing position, its spokesmen generally phrase their opposition in code words such as "impractical" or "an administrative nightmare." (This contention is refuted by the experience of the FEHBP and the Minneapolis–St. Paul employers.) Alternatively, industry spokesmen say they would want to be sure that the choices offered are *real* choices. I take this to mean that it is acceptable to require employers to offer HMOs which are few in number, usually small, and under present conditions not likely to become a serious threat to commercial insurance. But it is not acceptable to make insurers compete with each other in the same employee groups.

The industry view is that there is too much competition now. Therefore its members seek an antitrust exemption to allow them to band together to negotiate with providers over fees and charges. In fact, there is a great deal of competition in health insurance. Insurers compete with each other and with employer self-funded insurance for the exclusive business of an employer. But since all plans insure for essentially the same services from the same providers, they compete only on their administrative costs. They are virtually powerless to control which services are rendered, so they have almost no control over total costs. Only competition among providers offers hope of producing less costly styles of care, and competition among insurers does not create competition among providers.

The industry favors public utility regulation of hospitals in the form of certificate-of-need controls on capital investment and federal or state controls on hospital rates and budgets. It not only endorses existing control systems, but also recommends legislation to extend controls and make them more pervasive. For example, commercial insurers favor linking the certificate-of-need process to mandatory state prospective rate/budget review control systems. Aetna Life and Casualty and the Health Insurance Association of America recently have been running advertisements in national magazines endorsing health planning through Health Systems Agencies and state hospital rate review programs.

One reason the health insurance industry favors state rate regulation is because its members see in it an opportunity to secure equality among payors. Medicare and Medicaid today often reimburse less than the hospitals' full costs. And in some states Blue Cross's strong market position and historical relationship with hospitals enable Blue Cross to obtain a substantial discount. The result is that the hospitals make up the difference by higher charges to private-paying patients, the beneficiaries of the insurance companies, putting the insurance companies at a competitive disadvantage.

There are exceptions to the industry position. Some insurance companies are innovating and positioning themselves to be able to succeed in a competitive world. One of the most notable examples is SAFECO Life Insurance Company of Seattle which has developed a primary care network HMO in which participating physicians are paid a per-capita retainer fee for providing all office-based primary care services to enrolled patients and a cost control incentive payment for managing all their specialist and hospital care. Prudential has started group practice HMOs, and has even teamed up in Dallas with Kaiser-Permanente to create a new HMO there. Insurance Company of North America, which owns hospitals and HMOs, has testified forcefully in favor of economic competition.

Blue Cross/Blue Shield

The Blue Cross/Blue Shield Association is a trade association representing 143 independent not-for-profit Blue Cross and Blue Shield plans. There is a great variety in the history and market positions of these organizations, so one cannot easily generalize about them. However, Walter J. McNerney, President of the Blue Cross/Blue Shield National Association, has consistently testified in favor of the Federal Employees Health Benefits Program as a model for national health insurance.

One might wonder what differentiates Blue Cross/Blue Shield from the commercial insurance carriers. Both do most of their health insurance business on the basis of insured fee-for-service, a financing system whose share of the market would seem likely to decline with competition. However, insurance carriers have traditionally been quite remote from the providers of care and have paid for health services through indemnity payments and major medical insurance. In contrast, Blue Cross and Blue Shield were sponsored, respectively, by hospital and medical associations. And although they have gradually become more independent of provider control, they have remained much more deeply involved with providers. While competition would reduce the market share of insured fee-for-service, Blue Cross/Blue Shield could more easily develop alternative delivery systems than could commercial insurers. In fact, the Blues are now participating in about sixty-six alternative delivery system developments, and for this reason Blue Cross/Blue Shield leaders see themselves as likely to succeed in a competitive system.

CONCLUSION

In view of the reactions of these interest groups, what is the likely fate of proposals to create competition? The comprehensive proposal (CCHP) is not likely to be enacted all at once, since government tends to work incrementally, not in bold steps. The likely practical significance of CCHP will be as a guide or goal for incremental proposals which have a much better chance of enactment. As noted, the government is under severe fiscal pressure to control health care costs. This pressure is sure to become more intense in the coming years with increasing taxpayer resistance to the large and growing costs of health care, the need for large tax cuts for industry to encourage productive investment, the need to counter the Soviet military buildup, and other demands. The regulatory approach has been ineffective. The government can either try competition or wait until things get so bad that it can develop sufficient political support for the thoroughgoing controls advocated by Senator Kennedy and organized labor. While labor would prefer the latter, the hospitals and physicians would not.

Faced with an inescapable choice between tight government regulation or economic competition in the private sector, hospitals and physicians must find competition in their best interest. The reason is not because they would make more money under competition; they would probably make less. The reason is that it would enable them to avoid federal controls that would drastically curtail their freedom. It also seems likely that business leaders will prefer not to see such a large sector of the economy fall under federal controls.

At the time the Federal Employees Health Benefits Program was being considered by Congress, each of the interested groups had its own ideas as to what the program should look like. What finally emerged was a compromise that all groups could accept. It happened to be a model of fair market choice and competition. That such a program could simultaneously embody rational economic principles and a workable political compromise inspires some optimism about its potential as a model for universal health insurance.

11

LEWIS THOMAS

Your Very
Good Health*

Health care—the new name for medicine. The ideal health-care delivery system —what does it offer and who needs it? The doctor and his family. Most things get better by themselves. Computers v. common sense.

We spend $80 billion a year on health, as we keep reminding ourselves, or is it now $90 billion? Whichever, it is a shocking sum and just to mention it is to suggest the presence of a vast, powerful enterprise, intricately organized and coordinated. It is, however, a bewildering, essentially scatterbrained kind of busi-

*Reprinted with the author's permission from *The Lives of a Cell* (New York: Viking Press, 1974), pp. 81-86.

ness, expanding steadily without being planned or run by anyone in particular. Whatever sum we spent last year was only discovered after we'd spent it, and nobody can be sure what next year's bill will be. The social scientists, attracted by problems of this magnitude, are beginning to swarm in from all quarters to take a closer look and the economists are all over the place, pursing their lips and shaking their heads, shipping more and more data off to the computers, trying to decide whether this is a proper industry or a house of IBM cards. There doesn't seem to be any doubt about the amount of money being spent, but it is less certain where it goes, and for what.

It has become something of a convenience to refer to the whole endeavor as the "Health Industry." This provides the illusion that it is in a general way all one thing, and that it turns out, on demand, a single, unambiguous product, which is health. Thus, health care has become the new name for medicine. Health-care delivery is what doctors now do, along with hospitals and the other professionals who work with doctors, now known collectively as the health providers. The patients have become health consumers. Once you start on this line, there's no stopping. Just recently, to correct some of the various flaws, inequities, logistic defects, and near bankruptcies in today's health-care delivery system, the government has officially invented new institutions called Health Maintenance Organizations, already known familiarly as HMOs, spreading out across the country like post offices, ready to distribute in neat packages, as though from a huge, newly stocked inventory, health.

Sooner or later we are bound to get into trouble with this word. It is too solid and unequivocal a term to be used as a euphemism and this seems to be what we are attempting. I am worried that we may be overdoing it, taxing its meaning, to conceal an unmentionable reality that we've somehow agreed not to talk about in public. It won't work. Illness and death still exist and cannot be hidden. We are still beset by plain diseases, and we do not control them; they are loose on their own, afflicting us unpredictably and haphazardly. We are only able to deal with them when they have made their appearance, and we must use the methods of medical care for this as best we can, for better or worse.

It would be a better world if this were not true, but the fact is that diseases do not develop just because of carelessness about the preservation of health. We do not become sick only because of a failure of vigilance. Most illnesses, especially the major ones, are blind accidents that we have no idea how to prevent. We are really not all that good at preventing disease or preserving health—not yet anyway—and we are not likely to be until we have learned a great deal about disease mechanisms.

There is disagreement on this point, of course. Some of the believers among us are convinced that once we get a health-care delivery system that really works, the country might become a sort of gigantic spa which offers, like the labels on European mineral water bottles, preventives for everything from weak kidneys to moroseness.

It is a surprise that we haven't already learned that the word is a fallible incantation. Several decades of mental health have not made schizophrenia go away, nor has it been established that a community mental health center can yet maintain the mental health of a community. These admirable institutions are demonstrably useful for the management of certain forms of mental disease, but this is another matter.

My complaint about the terms is that they sound too much like firm promises. A Health Maintenance Organization, if well organized and financed, will have the best features of a clinic and hospital and should be of value to any community, but the people will expect it to live up to its new name. It will become, with the sign over its door, an official institution for the distribution of health, and if intractable heart disease develops in anyone thereafter, as it surely will (or multiple sclerosis, or rheumatoid arthritis, or the majority of cancers that can neither be prevented nor cured, or chronic nephritis, or stroke, or moroseness), the people will begin looking sidelong and asking questions in a low voice.

Meanwhile we are paying too little attention and respect to the built-in durability and sheer power of the human organism. Its surest tendency is toward stability and balance. It is a distortion, with something profoundly disloyal about it, to picture the human being as a teetering, fallible contraption always needing watching and patching, always on the verge of flapping to pieces; this is the doctrine that people hear most often and most eloquently on all our information media. We ought to be developing a much better system for general education about human health with more curricular time for acknowledgment, and even some celebration, of the absolute marvel of good health that is the real lot of most of us most of the time.

The familiar questions about the needs of the future in medicine are still before us. What items should be available, optimally, in an ideal health-care delivery system? How do you estimate the total need, per patient per year, for doctors, nurses, drugs, laboratory tests, hospital beds, X-rays, and so forth, in the best of rational worlds? My suggestion for a new way to develop answers is to examine in detail the ways in which the various parts of today's medical-care technology are used from one day to the next by the most sophisticated, knowledgeable, and presumably satisfied consumers who now have full access to the system—namely, the well-trained, experienced, middle-aged, married-with-family internists.

I could design the questionnaire myself, I think. How many times in the last five years have the members of your family, including yourself, had any kind of laboratory test? How many complete physical examinations? X-rays? Electrocardiograms? How often, in a year's turning, have you prescribed antibiotics of any kind for yourself or your family? How many hospitalizations? How much surgery? How many consultations with a psychiatrist? How many formal visits to a doctor, any doctor, including yourself?

I will bet that if you got this kind of information, and added everything up, you would find a quite different set of figures from the ones now being projected in official circles for the population at large. I have tried it already, in an unscientific way, by asking around among my friends. My data, still soft but fairly consistent, reveal that none of my internist friends have had a routine physical examination since military service; very few have been X-rayed except by dentists; almost all have resisted surgery; laboratory tests for anyone in the family are extremely rare. They use a lot of aspirin, but they seem to write very few prescriptions and almost never treat family fever with antibiotics. This is not to say that they do not become ill; these families have the same incidence of chiefly respiratory and gastrointestinal illness as everyone else, the same number of anxieties and bizarre notions, and the same number—on balance, a small number—of frightening or devastating diseases.

It will be protested that internists and their households are really full-time captive patients and cannot fairly be compared to the rest of the population. As each member of the family appears at the breakfast table the encounter is, in effect, a house call. The father is, in the liveliest sense, a family doctor. This is true, but all the more reason for expecting optimal use to be made of the full range of medicine's technology. There is no problem of access; the entire health-care delivery system is immediately at hand, and the cost of all items is surely less than that for nonmedical families. All the usual constraints that limit the use of medical care by the general population are absent.

If my hunch, based on the small sample of professional friends, is correct, these people appear to use modern medicine quite differently from the ways in which we have systematically been educating the public over the last few decades. It cannot be explained away as an instance of shoemakers' children going without shoes. Doctors' families do tend to complain that they receive less medical attention than their friends and neighbors, but they seem a normal, generally healthy lot with a remarkably low incidence of iatrogenic illness.

The great secret, known to internists and learned early in marriage by internists' wives but still hidden from the general public, is that most things get better by themselves. Most things, in fact, are better by morning.

It is conceivable that we might be able to provide good medical care for everyone needing it in a new system designed to assure equity, provided we can restrain ourselves or our computers from designing a system in which all 200 million of us are assumed to be in constant peril of failed health every day of our lives. In the same sense that our judicial system presumes us to be innocent until proved guilty, a medical-care system may work best if it starts with the presumption that most people are healthy. Left to themselves, computers may try to do it in the opposite way, taking it as given that some sort of direct, continual, professional intervention is required all the time to maintain the health of each citizen, and we will end up spending all our money on nothing but that. Meanwhile there is a long list of other things to do if we are to change the way we live together—especially in our cities—in time. Social health is another kind of problem, more complex and urgent, and there will be other bills to pay.

12

COTTON M. LINDSAY

Recapitulation and Coda

NHI and nationalization—the fallacies of distinguishing between them. Political and economic problems inherent to government displacement of medical markets. Deep and shallow insurance coverage. The costs of various NHI proposals. Consumer choice health plan. The need for caution.

The desirability of national health insurance (NHI) in any form must be demonstrated in terms of stated objectives. It is remarkable at this late date, with broad bipartisan support in Congress for some sort of legislation in this area, that those objectives can be so vague. Most advocates of NHI couch their arguments in terms of glib and rather vacuous phrases such as "introducing planning and imposing rationality on the system" or "eliminating duplication and redundancy of function." These phrases describe *means*, not objectives. Planning is useful only if planned resource use produces preferred results and eliminating duplication is desirable only if the reduction in the quality and quantity of output are worth less than the resources freed.

It is clear that an objective which is *not* served by national health insurance is health itself. As Dr. Kass points out in the opening chapter, there is little evidence that even the most generous bill under consideration will influence the nation's health. Adult health as indicated by such indexes as life expectancy responded rather insignificantly to the introduction of all the medical miracles of the twentieth century. Changing the manner in which we pay for these miracles can hardly be expected to have a profound effect. Kass mentions, however, that individuals may make quite dramatic effects on their health by simply initiating small changes in their lifestyles—by giving up smoking and by eating moderately. The unwillingness of most people to take these small steps says a great deal about the value which members of the public place on marginal health increments. Congress should bear this revealed valuation in mind when it considers committing large amounts of taxpayers' money to provide medical care people would not provide for themselves—and which is unproductive in any event. The tenuous connection between health and health care is reemphasized by Lewis Thomas's observation concerning the frequency with which doctors themselves (and their families) see other doctors.

The implicit intent of national health insurance may simply be to redistribute income from rich to poor or, according to Schelling (Chapter 2), from the rich to those who would be made poor by the expenses associated with a catastrophic illness. If this is its function, then we must recognize that avoidance of such financial calamities is the province of private health insurance. The desirability of NHI must in this event be weighed against the observation that nearly everyone is already covered against such losses by either private health insurance, Medicare, or Medicaid. It should also be noted that in shifting the organizational nexus of health insurance from the private sector to the government we do not automatically eliminate or even reduce its cost. We simply pay these bills as taxpayers rather than as insurance subscribers.

Proponents of NHI are quick to draw the distinction that it is national health insurance they favor—not nationalization of the industry such as occurred under the British National Health Service. Seldon (Chapter 3) illustrates in detail the fallacies in such a distinction. First, it is the absence of price as a rationing mechanism and guide to resource allocation which is responsible for most of the problems of the National Health Service— not the fact that it is "owned" by the government. As price would serve neither of these functions under most of the proposed legislation currently before Congress, the fact that resources remain in the private sector with NHI fails to redeem any of these proposals. Second, Seldon indicates that national health insurance brings with it the seeds of eventual nationalization. The demand for care by the public, freed from the constraint of paying fees for each service, spirals upward, causing prices and governmental budget obligations to soar. In an attempt to get control over costs, government begins to regulate suppliers by curbing investment and putting ceilings on prices. These have the effect of making the industry unattractive to potential investors of both physical and human capital. Thus eventual nationalization may be difficult to avoid.

Seldon notes that Great Britain already had a national health insurance program when it adopted the National Health Service in 1946. The Canadian system, often held up as an example to the United States of a model upon which NHI should be based, is already exhibiting symptoms of the problems which Seldon foresees. Controls and ceilings on physician fees have already been imposed and investment is being curtailed. Deterioration in the quality of service cannot be far behind.

Empirical analysis of experience under both the older model, the British National Health Service, and the newer variant in Canada supports Seldon's contentions. In these systems, displacement of markets in allocation of care has not rationalized these activities. Chapter 4 shows that the ability of government to plan is tempered on the one hand by the technical difficulty of the task and on the other by the political forces which inevitably are brought to bear on government budgetary decisions.

The Canadian NHI, for example, relies on a reimbursement system which has increased the geographic imbalance of physicians across Canada. Similar results were produced by introduction of the NHS in Great Britain. To these technical problems associated with planning, however, we must add the influence of politics. Significant evidence of political manipulation of NHS spending by the party in power in the English parliament was also reported there.

A third problem with government displacement of markets in an area like health is that no one has an incentive to economize. Not only do people behave as though health care costs them nothing when they demand it, it becomes very difficult for them to determine how much it does in fact cost them or anyone else. Econometric analysis discussed in Chapter 4 reveals that the adoption of NHI in Canada effectively shifted much of the cost of medical care for the nation onto the shoulders of the economically disadvantaged. Introduction of NHI there was accompanied by restraints on welfare spending which made possible the large budgetary outlays for this program without increased taxation.

Another possible objective of national health insurance may be to increase the efficiency with which medical care is supplied. In Chapter 5 we address the question of how effectively existing institutions providing physician care have supplied the market for these services. We seek to discover, specifically, whether problems peculiar to the medical care industry have caused the industry to perform less than adequately, suggesting the desirability of national health insurance to promote efficiency. We have analyzed and rejected each of these arguments. The argument that government health care would better provide the people's health needs is considered in light of a detailed study of health statistics of Canada, England, and the United States.

These health indicators fail to reveal any impact of the introduction of government health initiatives in any of the three countries considered.

It is true and widely recognized that consumers of medical care are at a severe disadvantage when they face physicians on the opposite side of market transactions. Physicians know whether their services are likely to be productive; even after the treatments have been performed, patients frequently are unable to determine that productivity. The important question is not whether this problem exists, but rather what is the best way to organize the provision of medical care in response to it. We argue in Chapter 5 that no system is demonstrably superior to the present pluralistic scheme which leaves the organization of medical services to private investors.

This Panglosian view does not extend to the insurance and hospital sector. Although everyone has some form of hospitalization insurance, much of that insurance is "shallow," while coverage of catastrophic losses is most logical from an economist's point of view. Second, the cost-reimbursement type of insurance typically associated with nonprofit "Blue" plans encourages waste and excessive capitalization of nonprofit voluntary hospitals. Both of these problems will likely cure themselves. Private insurance has experienced phenomenal growth in the postwar period, rising from virtually nothing to over 80 percent of the population in thirty years. It seems reasonable to expect that, as experience accumulates with the various formulas, individual understanding of the wisdom of "deep" coverage will influence people to demand this in their plans.

The late arrival of the superior indemnity insurance in the market has not prevented it from experiencing even faster growth and capturing a significant and increasing share of this market. Indemnity insurance, by relying on the payment of flat fees for medical exigencies such as "a hospital day," provides incentives for patients and their physicians to seek out economical hospitals which avoid waste and the higher prices associated with it. As private insurers are able to offer such plans at considerable savings over the waste-prone "Blues," they can be expected to continue owing at the expense of less efficient plans. As larger and larger numbers of hospital service demanders come to be covered by indemnity insurance and thus become more cost-conscious, the competitive pressure on hospitals—even on nonprofit hospitals—to cut costs and eliminate waste will mount.

Jack Meyer surveys the plethora of NHI proposals currently before Congress (Chapter 8). These range from the comprehensive (and costly) administration and Kennedy bills to the more modest Durenberger, Ullman, and Schweiker proposals. While the former seek to involve the government in every aspect of health care industry organization, the latter seek primarily to provide tax and other economic incentives for more efficient private sector organization of this activity.

Meyer's analysis of the cost of these proposals is particularly useful. He points out that most discussions of costs ignore substantial elements of cost. In most estimates, attention is focused on the budgetary cost of NHI to the federal government and disregards the fact that many of the more elaborate proposals mandate substantial increases in health insurance contributions by employers and wage earners. As budgetary costs alone for the Kennedy bill are projected to be over $200 billion, the magnitude of these hidden costs has not even been estimated by the administration or other sponsors of the legislation. Glib reference to hospital cost containment and negotiated fees would lead us to believe that such costs will be unimportant. The discussion by Congressmen Stockman and Gramm (Chapter 6) attests eloquently to the sort of cost relief we may expect from this source.

Phelps (Chapter 7) reviews the scope and experience that the United States has had with government financing and provision of medical care. He finds that government is already financing—through subsidies to the purchase, supply, or in the form of tax deductions—more than half the cost of health care in the United States. He also notes that the existing Medicare and Medicaid programs have been quite successful at increasing utilization among the elderly and the poor. The number of hospital days of care per person consumed by the elderly increased by nearly 50 percent under Medicare. Although ardent centralizers have expressed considerable unhappiness with the decentralized Medicaid program, Phelps is also able to show that Medicaid has been quite successful in leveling coverage and utilization of care across income groups. For example, the strong negative correlation between income and physician visits per year which existed before Medicaid has been successfully reversed. The most intensive users of physician services in 1973 were those persons with incomes under $3,000 per year and the next most intensive users were those with incomes between $3,000 and $7,000 per year.

Phelps notes that employment status explains virtually all of the remaining lack of coverage for individuals with earnings of more than $7,000. This suggests that the largest "hole" in the present network of coverage is medical insurance for those who lose their employer-sponsored group insurance when they become unemployed. He also notes that a strong inducement to purchase private medical insurance is the deductibility of these premiums on federal income tax. Because of the progressivity of the rate structure, the size of the subsidy rises rapidly with income. For example, someone with an income of only $3,000 per year receives a subsidy of $48 toward his medical insurance coverage while a person earning in excess of $50,000 receives a subsidy of $362.

In Chapter 9, Leffler and I report estimates made in 1976 of the long-run effect of national health insurance on the supply and prices of medical care. Two plans were considered. Under the so-called moderate plan an eventual increase of 12 percent occurs in the quantity of physicians, and fees rise only moderately—in real terms, increasing by a maximum of 42 percent. In contrast, a complete plan such as the old Corman-Kennedy proposal would produce an eventual 23 percent increase in the number of physicians, but the cost would be staggering. Because the plan would be implemented fully in the first year, physician fees are predicted to rise 277 percent, producing an average income of $168,000 in that first year. Both plans would benefit from over-adjustment to the demand shock of Medicare and Medicaid, which caused the rate of entry into medical practice to exceed the expected increase in demand for physician services. Without these plans physician fees are actually expected to decline over the near term.

Since we first made these calculations, legislative proposals have changed and presumably the numbers are all larger. (It is not clear how much larger. Our original calculations were made in real, inflation-adjusted, 1975 dollars.) Even though the proposals have changed in their details, the same problems exist with the new proposals.

Congress will not tolerate fee increases such as those predicted for the complete plan. Indeed, many of the proposals already contain provisions for setting fee ceilings for physicians. Such controls over prices will have two effects. First, they will retard the adjustment of supply to the shortages produced by the subsidy aspects of the programs. Second, in the absence of rationing by price, some other form of rationing will have to be adopted. Almost certainly that form will be of the resource-using type such as waiting in queues. The resource waste associated with both effects has been estimated.

Because of the excess capacity in current physician output, the welfare cost associated with the adjustment of supply is negligible, reaching a maximum of only $783 million per year with the complete plan. In contrast, the waste associated with queuing or other resource-using rationing devices is predicted to reach a maximum of $17 billion per year and to average nearly $10 billion per year over the entire quarter of a century for which the forecasts were performed. Considering that the government and the private sector combined are currently spending only $22 billion per year on physician services, the magnitude of such waste is truly staggering. The numbers have probably increased since we first made our calculations, but the relationships are undoubtedly the same.

Government initiatives in the health area need not lead us down the path of skyrocketing inflation in health care cost controls and endless red tape to a destination characterized by bureaucratic indifference and mediocrity. Some of the proposals before Congress would lead us away from Canadian and British models in the direction of genuinely innovative change in the industry. Chapter 10 contains a description of such a plan: Alain Enthoven's consumer choice health plan, which would foster rather than suppress market forces in the medical care sector. Such a plan would eliminate current barriers to the introduction of prepaid group plans by requiring that employees selecting an employer-based group plan would have to bear the full cost, choosing a more costly fee for a service type arrangement.

Whether the American medical care consumer will ultimately opt for care provided under these circumstances remains to be seen. That prepaid plans can reduce costs is clear. Whether the cost reductions are purchased with an excessive loss of independence and personal attention can only be determined by those who are enrolled. This choice can be made efficiently when fee for service and prepaid care compete on an equal footing. Consumer choice health plan makes such a choice possible.

Most of us already have private insurance with quite high limits. Some of us should probably increase our coverage to extend to the rare catastrophic event which might otherwise ruin us financially. The latter problem is primarily an educational one—not unlike the task of influencing us to eat well and less, a program likely to be far more productive healthwise. Most of the rest of us are covered by the generous Medicare and Medicaid programs. The small holes in this network of coverage may require patches of about the same magnitude. They do not warrant a major bureaucratic overhaul of the health industry. This industry has performed well in adapting to rapidly changing technology and in providing care of high quality to a broad spectrum of demanders. Under the circumstances, we should exercise the greatest caution in imposing changes on either the financing or delivery methods of this faithful servant.

NOTES

1. Leon R. Kass: "Medical Care and the Pursuit of Health"

1. During the period between 1900 and 1970, among white males in the United States the average life expectancy calculated from increased by about 22 years, the biggest contribution being a decline in infant mortality; for those who reached age sixty-five the average life expectancy increased only 1.5 years.

2. A recent lawsuit in Maryland illustrates how consumerism and governmental participation can work together toward this result. A married woman brought suit against two Washington suburban hospitals that refused to permit her to undergo voluntary sterilization procedures in their facilities, even though her physician agreed to perform the operation. One hospital had refused permission on moral grounds, the other because the patient and her husband refused to comply with hospital regulations for sterilization procedures that required permission of the spouse. The suit claimed that the hospitals, because they had received Hill-Burton funding for construction, were obliged to meet the health needs of all members of the community without discrimination. What was blithely assumed by the plaintiff was that the community, or rather each member thereof, is the final judge of what constitutes a *health need*.

3. Dr. Lee is a former assistant secretary for health at HEW.

4. Cotton M. Lindsay, Arthur Seldon: "More Evidence on Britain and Canada"

1. It was found that waiting time for an appointment in Quebec increased on average from six to eleven days immediately after CNHI began. This occurred although the number of physicians in Quebec was increasing rapidly at that time.

2. This is not to say that *delay* itself is costless. On the contrary, delay plays an important role in the analysis. Delay may mean inability to work and function due to the crippling effects of disease and injury. The difference is that these costs do not ration in the way that waiting costs ration in the waiting room. The higher the cost of delay in restoring productivity and normal healthy activity, the *more* eagerly will hospitalization be sought.

3. A statistical model based on this interpretation was estimated. Coefficients of relevant variables in these regressions all the predicted signs and were highly significant. The equation explained 30 percent of the variation in mean waiting times for a selected sample of diseases across hospital regions (Lindsay 1979).

4. Rates of return represent the interest rate that would make the earnings of general practitioners just as attractive as those of other careers. If this rate is lower than rates earned in other careers, it implies that doctors suffer financially by becoming doctors. Henderson-Stewart in an appendix to Blaug (1965) estimates a rate of return of 14 percent for all higher education. Layard et al. (1971) report a rate of 12 percent. Ziderman (1971) concludes that this rate is 20 percent.

5. The latest estimate, made in December 1979 by a leading figure in the British Medical Association, Anthony Grabham, envisaged waiting lists for hospitals at a million patients. The figure for March 1979 was 750,000.

5. Cotton M. Lindsay: "The Organization of Medical Care Markets"

1. This is not to say that medical need has *never* been incorporated into economic analysis. See, for example, the imaginative treatment by Culyer (1979). Most analysis merely stops when need is introduced, however, with the observation that such considerations may obviate conventional arguments based on efficiency.

2. In my study of the British NHS, a model of queuing by list is developed in which rationing involves no sacrifice of the demanders' time. Instead, the queue is simply allowed to grow until the wait for care itself produces an equilibrium, i.e., until the number joining equals the number treated. Such a queue rations on the basis of the longevity of the condition. Those who will no longer need the care by the time it can be delivered are crowded out by chronic cases which do not respond to self-treatment. Data on NHS waiting lists for hospitals were analyzed for the presence of this sort of rationing, and its presence was conclusively confirmed. See Lindsay (1979), Chapter 3.

3. In Leffler and Lindsay (1978) the effect of all subsidies taken together is estimated to reduce the market price of physician care by more than 50 percent below its "full cost" level.

4. Capture of the Civil Aeronautics Board by airlines to promote monopolistic airfares on scheduled routes is a well-known example; another is the cosy relationship between truckers and the Interstate Commerce Commission. Public utility commissions, milk marketing, and alcoholic control boards are slightly less familiar examples.

5. Similarly, the same ignorance on the part of consumers which leads them to surrender their control over *how much* care they demand from the market has been alleged to bias the mix of services they obtain. They are seen as underinvesting in prevention and devoting most of their care dollars for treatment. The proverb which holds that "an ounce of prevention is worth a pound of cure" may have been true given the actual therapeutic and preventive options available in Benjamin Franklin's day, but exchange rates vary over time. There is considerable doubt—among those analysts who have actually costed out the resources consumed and the value of the diagnoses and treatment provided—that health "screening" and related medical care aimed at prevention is actually cost effective. See Schweitzer (1974), pp. 22–32.

6. David A. Stockman, W. Philip Gramm: "The Administration's Case for Hospital Cost Containment"

1. More highly trained, skilled staff, specialty-intensive care units (coronary, burn, neonatal), and more sophisticated diagnostic and treatment methods and technologies.

2. For example, a recent cost-benefit analysis by the College of American Pathologists demonstrated that mechanizing an annual volume of 32,000 lab tests resulted in a net cost decrease for such tests of 16.7 percent annually.

7. Charles E. Phelps: "Public Sector Medicine: History and Analysis"

1. Mitchell and Vogel (1975) reported tax expenditures for direct medical care payments of $1.3 billion for 1970. The medical care component of the CPI has risen by approximately 80 percent since then, indicating that the analogous figure for 1980 would be $2.5 billion.

2. To provide an indication of the rates of growth in these more hidden components of government intervention in medical care, consider the case of the tax subsidy to employer-paid health insurance premiums. In 1970 this subsidy was estimated to be $1.6 billion. By 1975 the estimate had grown to $5.5 billion, although revised estimates now make that amount closer to $7 billion. The rapid growth in employer premium payments has increased the tax subsidy to $13 billion by 1980 (Phelps 1980).

3. The magnitude of the intergenerational transfer is assessed in Browning (1973).

4. In FY 1975, hospital payments for 23 million aged and disabled persons were $10.7 billion.

5. Premium payments of $80.40 per year by enrollees represent 39 percent of Part B revenues (Mueller and Gibson 1976).

6. For a more extensive analysis of this phenomenon, see Newhouse (1976), particularly the Appendix.

7. Many private health insurance policies for persons under sixty-five now have true catastrophic provisions included, wherein insurance coverage becomes complete once out-of-pocket payments have exceeded some fixed amount (e.g., $1,000).

8. See Andersen et al. (1972) for a description of this study.

9. When demand is price-inelastic, total expenditure rises with price. If demand is price-elastic, expenditure would fall as price increased, because quantities purchased would fall more than enough to offset price increases.

10. Primarily for this reason, fewer and fewer doctors accept Medicare payment assignment, since by so doing they agree to accept that amount as payment in full for services rendered.

11. Leffler and Lindsay discuss this problem at greater length in Chapter 9.

12. Being married to a physician, I view such a result with more mixed emotions than the typical patient-consumer.

13. These estimates are from Mitchell and Phelps (1976) and Phelps (1980).

14. For hospitalization, the patient pays $25 per stay or $3.50 per day, whichever is larger. For other care there is an annual deductible amount of $50 to $100, beyond which the patient pays either 20 or 25 percent of all charges.

15. I have benefited from discussions with David S. C. Chu and Susan Hosek of The Rand Corporation in formulating this section, although the usual phrases absolving them of responsibility for my errors should hold more than usually in this case.

16. Under the Berry Plan, physicians were allowed to complete their residency training before their service duty and were guaranteed a service position matching their specialty training. Since many physicians had signed Berry Plan agreements before the end of the draft, their commitments to the military may have begun several years past the end of the Vietnam War.

17. In the latter case, if firms price at marginal cost, revenues will not meet average costs and the firm is unprofitable. Either the product will not be produced privately, or a higher price will be set and "too little" produced.

8. Jack A. Meyer: "Proposals under Consideration"

1. This assumes that the marginal cost of incremental units of health care rises as additional units are provided, an assumption which seems reasonable for a service like medical care provided by factors of production whose supply is apt to be quite scarce. See Hall (1976b), pp. 167–69.

2. For an elaboration of the details of this plan, see HEW (1979). Also see the administration's proposed legislation—S. 1812, 96th Congress, 1st session.

3. Press release, Senator Edward M. Kennedy, 14 May 1979, p. 1.

4. Ibid.

5. See press release, Senator Dave Durenberger, July 1977, p. 4.

6. Durenberger's proposal stipulates that at least two of the three plans must be "alternative health plans (that stimulate competition), if available."

7. See HEW (1979). Actual total spending, including those services not covered by NHP, is likely to be roughly $230 billion in FY 1980.

8. Other categories of projected federal expenditures include $2.1 billion for administration expense, $1.6 billion for subsidized care for low-wage or high-risk workers, $0.5 billion for Health Care fund coverage of those who do not fall into the employment, aged, disabled, or poverty groups, and $(−0.6) billion for tax effects.

9. Currently, part-time workers are about 20 percent of the size of the group working full time. Since HEW estimates that it will cost employers $6.1 billion to cover full-time workers, one could begin by estimating that it would cost another $1.2 billion to cover the part-time work force (20 percent of $6.1 billion). However, about three-fourths of the part-time workers are classified as working part-time for economic reasons, the other one-fourth working part-time voluntarily, and many people in the former category are likely to be more expensive to cover than the average worker. In other words, the part-time work force probably has a disproportionate share of people with above-average health expenditures. Thus, an estimate of $1.5 billion for covering this group might be more realistic.

10. For an analysis of the increase in hospital costs and the initial legislative proposals to restrict the rate of increase, see American Enterprise Institute (1978). For an analysis of more recent proposals to contain hospital costs, see CBO (1979a).

11. Includes small savings from FY 1979.

12. The CBO estimate of $11.3 billion in 1984 savings is comprised of $4.1 billion and $0.62 billion in reduced Medicare and Medicaid payments, respectively, and $6.6 billion of nonfederal savings. These figures are lower than those reported earlier by CBO, reflecting updated projections.

13. Furthermore, the CBO report (1979a) states that their own estimates may be too high due to such factors as offsets arising from increased outpatient expenditures (not accounted for in the CBO estimates), exceptions granted by HEW, and possible evasion techniques employed by hospitals, such as spinning off various hospital functions (see pp. 29–30). The lower CBO estimates result primarily from different assumptions about the response of hospital behavior to the bill, but are also affected by different assumptions about inflation, hospital expenditures, and hospital admissions.

14. For an examination of the available evidence concerning HMO performance, see Luft (1979).

15. For an explanation of the advantages of such variety, see McClure (1978).

16. *Congressional Record*, vol. 125, no. 112, 96th Congress, 1st session (6 September 1979), p. 61.

17. See, for example, Salkever and Bice (1979), and Sloan and Steinwald (1978).

9. Keith B. Leffler, Cotton M. Lindsay: "The Long-Run Effects of National Health Insurance on Medical Care Prices and Output"

1. The effects of Medicare and Medicaid in this respect are well documented. See, e.g., Feldstein (1970a), Sloan (1976), and Cashin (1970).

2. Some have argued further that the stock of physicians itself influences demand through physicians' advice to patients regarding follow-up visits and additional clinical procedures. Our empirical evidence reported in this chapter, however, does not support this hypothesis. This view is reported in Sloan (1976).

3. Chapter 5 elaborates on this point.

4. For example, see Freeman (1975) for a model of producing similar results for Ph.D. training of scientific personnel.

5. This may be clarified by reference to Figure 3. At any given time there is a fixed stock of physicians with an associated earnings level which clears the market. For example, given an existing stock of physicians S_T and the demand curve, earnings will be E_T. There is also a level of earnings that we may calculate which would just compensate physicians for the years of investment in training. Assume that to be E_O. If demand conditions did not change, we would expect the stock of physicians to expand until earnings fell to that level; hence the long-run equilibrium stock in Figure 3 is S_O. The difference in this long-run equilibrium (optimal) stock S_O and the actual stock S_T is what we refer to here as the physician shortage.

7. See Lindsay et al. (1976), Chapter 4, for the statistical evidence on this point and an extended discussion.

8. One response, of course, could be a lowering of standards. This could necessitate a change in state licensing standards. We neglect this alternative as unlikely.

9. Since time is less valuable to some demanders than others, in general a different population will receive care via queuing than obtains it with price rationing. Those who place a low value on their time will be willing to outwait those whose time has valuable alternative uses. This should have only a negligible effect on its value, however.

10. The estimates of the potential social waste through nonprice rationing were calculated assuming all physicians are in private practice, averaging the same number of patient visits as general practitioners. (This number is assumed to be 8,160 per year as reported in *Medical Economics*, a manual continuing survey.) This serves to overstate the number of actual visits but understates the expected waiting time, i.e., both the implicit price and valuations would be proportionally higher in Tables 4 and 10. To the extent that interspecialty decisions are rationally made on pecuniary grounds, there should be no net bias in the estimates of Tables 9 and 10.

11. See Lindsay (1969), pp. 351–62, for an economic interpretation of this view as well as some cautionary footnotes.

12. All dollar variables in constant (1956–1958 = 1.00) dollars. All T statistics in parentheses. All R^2s corrected for degree of freedom.

13. See Lindsay et al. (1976), Chapter 2, for a complete discussion of this estimation.

REFERENCES

American Enterprise Institute. 1978. *Proposals for the Regulation of Hospital Costs* (8 June). Washington, DC: American Enterprise Institute for Public Policy Research.

American Hospital Association. 1975. *American Hospital Association Guide to the Health Care Field.* Chicago: American Hospital Association.

———. 1979. *American Hospital Association Guide to the Health Care Field: 1979 Edition.* Chicago: American Hospital Association.

Andersen, Ronald, et al. 1972. *Health Service Use: National Trends and Variations—1953–1971.* Washington, DC: U.S. Department of Health, Education, and Welfare.

Belloc, Nedra B. 1973. "Relationship of Health Practices and Mortality." *Preventive Medicine* 2:67–81.

———, and Breslow, Lester. 1972. "Relationship of Physical Health Status and Health Practices." *Preventive Medicine* 1:409–21.

Berger, Emile, and Mosberg, William Jr. 1979. "Ten Years of National Health Service in Canada." *Neurosurgery* 4, 6.

Berki, Sylvester E. 1972. *Hospital Economics.* Lexington, MA: Heath Publishing Company.

Blaug, M. 1965. "The Rate of Return on Investment in Education in Great Britain." *The Manchester School* (September).

Browning, Edgar K. 1973. "Social Insurance and Intergenerational Transfers." *Journal of Law and Economics* 16 (October):215–38.

Cashin, J., ed. 1970. *The Impact of the Advent of Medicare on Hospital Costs.* Hempstead, NY: Hofstra University.

Cocks, Douglas L., and Virts, John R. 1974. "Pricing Behavior of the Ethical Pharmaceutical Industry." *Journal of Business* 47, 3 (July):349–62.

Congressional Budget Office. 1979a. *Controlling Rising Hospital Costs* (September). Washington, DC: Congress of the United States.

———. 1979b. "Profile of Health Care Coverage: The Haves and Have-Nots." Washington, DC: Congress of the United States.

Cooper, Michael, and Culyer, Anthony J. 1970. *Health Services Financing.* London: British Medical Association.

Culyer, Anthony J. 1979. *Need and the National Health Service.* London: Martin Robertson.

Ellenbogen, Gladys. 1974. "Private Health Insurance Supplementary to Medicare." Working paper prepared for the Special Committee on Aging, U.S. Senate. Washington, DC: U.S. Government Printing Office.

Enterline, Philip E. 1973. "Effects of 'Free' Medical Care on Medical Practice—the Quebec Experience." *The New England Journal of Medicine* 288, 22 (31 May):1152–55.

———, et al. 1973. "The Distribution of Medical Services Before and After 'Free' Medical Care—the Quebec Experience." *The New England Journal of Medicine* 289, 22 (29 November):1174–78.

Enthoven, Alain C. 1979. "Consumer-Centered vs. Job-Centered Health Insurance." *Harvard Business Review* 57, 1 (January-February):141–52.

Feldstein, Martin. 1970*a*. "Hospital Cost Inflation: A Study of Nonprofit Price Dynamics." *The American Economic Review* (December).

———. 1970*b*. "The Rising Price of Physicians' Serices." *Review of Economics and Statistics* (May).

———. 1973. "The Welfare Cost of Excess Health Insurance." *Journal of Political Economy* 81 (March/April).Freeman, Richard. 1975. "Supply and Sal-

Freeman, Richard. 1975. "Supply and Salary Adjustments to the Changing Science Manpower Market: Physics, 1948–1973." *American Economic Review* (March).

Friedman, Milton, and Kuznets, Simon. 1945. *Income for Independent Professional Practice.* New York: National Bureau of Economic Research, Columbia University Press.

General Accounting Office. 1975. *Performance of the Social Security Administration Compared with That of Private Fiscal Intermediaries in Dealing with Institutional Providers.* Washington, DC: U.S. Government Printing Office.

Gibson, Robert M., and Fisher, Charles R. 1978. "National Health Expenditures, Fiscal Year 1977." *Social Security Bulletin* 41, 7 (July).

Hall, Thomas D. 1976*a*. "The Behavior of Hospitals as Nonprofit Firms." Doctoral dissertation, University of California at Los Angeles.

———. 1976*b*. "Proposals under Consideration." In Cotton M. Lindsay, ed., *New Directions in Public Health Care*, 2d ed. San Francisco: Institute for Contemporary Studies.

Institute of Medicine. 1973. *Disease by Disease toward National Health Insurance?* Washington, DC: Institute of Medicine, National Academy of Sciences.

Kass, Leon R. 1975. "Regarding the End of Medicine and the Pursuit of Health." *The Public Interest*, No. 40 (Summer).

Kessel, Reuben. 1970. "The AMA and the Supply of Physicians." *Law and Contemporary Problems* (Spring).

Layard, P. R. G., et al. 1971. *Qualified Manpower and Economic Performance.* London: Penguin.

Lee, Philip R., and Jonsen, Albert R. 1974. "Editorial: The Right to Health Care." *American Review of Respiratory Disease* 109:591–92.

Leffler, Keith B. 1977. "Competition and Monopoly in the Supply of Physician Services." Doctoral dissertation, University of California at Los Angeles.

———. 1978. "Physician Licensure: Competition and Monopoly in American Medicine." *Journal of Law and Economics* (April).

————, and Lindsay, Cotton M. 1978. "Student Discount Rates, Consumption Loans and Subsidies to Professional Education." UCLA Discussion Paper No. 132.

Lewis, H. G. 1963. *Unionism and Relative Wages in the United States.* Chicago: University of Chicago Press.

Lindsay, Cotton M. 1978. *Canadian National Health Insurance: Lessons for the United States.* Nutley, NJ: Roche Laboratories.

————. 1979. *Government in Medicine: The British Experience.* Nutley, NJ: Roche Laboratories.

————. 1969. "Medical Care and the Economics of Sharing." *Economica* (November).

————. 1973. "Real Returns to Medical Education." *Journal of Human Resources.*

————. 1976. "A Theory of Government Enterprise." *Journal of Political Economy* (October).

————. 1975. *Veterans Administration Hospitals: An Economic Analysis of Government Enterprise.* Washington, DC: American Enterprise Institute for Public Policy Research.

————, and Hall, Thomas D. 1980. "Medical Schools: Producers of What? Sellers to Whom?" *Journal of Law and Economics* (forthcoming).

————; Hall, Thomas D.; Leffler, Keith B; Munson, C. E. 1976. *The Medical Education Market: An Economic Analysis of the Behavior of Demanders and Suppliers of Medical Training.* Los Angeles: Professional Education Project, University of California at Los Angeles.

Luft, Harold S. 1979. "HMOs, Competition, Cost Containment, and NHI." In Mark V. Pauley, ed., *National Health Insurance: What Now, What Later, What Never?* Proceedings of American Enterprise Institute Conference, 4–5 October. Washington, DC: American Enterprise Institute for Public Policy Research.

McClure, Walter. 1978. "On Broadening the Definition of and Removing Regulatory Barriers to a Competitive Health Care System." *Journal of Health, Politics, and Law* 3, 3 (Fall).

Mitchell, Bridger M., and Phelps, Charles E. 1976. "National Health Insurance: Some Costs and Effects of Mandated Coverage." *Journal of Political Economy* 84 (June).

Mitchell, Bridger M., and Vogel, Ronald J. 1975. "Health and Taxes: An Assessment of the Medical Deduction." *Southern Economic Journal* 41 (April).

Morison, R. S. 1974. "Rights and Responsibilities: Redressing the Uneasy Balance." *The Hastings Center Report* 4, 2 (April):4.

Mueller, Marjorie Smith, and Gibson, Robert M. 1976. "National Health Expenditures, Fiscal Year 1975." *Social Security Bulletin* (February).

Newhouse, Joseph P. 1979. "The Geographic Distribution of Physicians: Is the Conventional Wisdom Correct?" Paper presented at December meetings of American Economics Association (Atlanta, Georgia).

———. 1976. "Health Care Cost Sharing and Cost Containment." Testimony before the U.S. House of Representatives Committee on Interstate Commerce, 24 February 1976. Duplicated. Santa Monica, CA: The Rand Corporation.

———, Phelps, Charles E., and Schwartz, William B. 1974. "Policy Options and the Impact of National Health Insurance." *New England Journal of Medicine* 290 (13 June).

Niskanen, William A. 1968. "Nonmarket Decision Making: The Peculiar Economics of Bureaucracy." *American Economic Review* 58 (May).

Pauly, Mark V., ed. 1980. *National Health Insurance: What Now, What Later, What Never?* Proceedings of American Enterprise Institute conference. Washington, DC: American Enterprise Institute for Public Policy Research.

Peltzman, Sam. 1976. "Toward a More General Theory of Regulation." *Journal of Law and Economics* 19 (August):211–40.

Phelps, Charles E. 1974. "The Distribution and Effectiveness of Private Health Insurance." Testimony before the U.S. House of Representatives Committee on Interstate Commerce. In *National Health Insurance—Implications.* Washington, DC: U.S. Government Printing Office.

———. 1975. "The Effects of Insurance on the Demand for Medical Care." In Ronald Andersen et al., eds., *Equity in Health Services: Empirical Analyses in Social Policy.* Cambridge, MA: Ballinger Publishing Company.

———. 1980. "National Health Insurance and Mandated Employee Benefits."In Mark V. Pauly, ed., *National Health Insurance: What Now, What Later, What Never?* Proceedings of American Enterprise Institute conference. Washington, DC: American Enterprise Institute for Public Policy Research.

Rayack, Elton. 1967. *Professional Power and American Medicine.* N.p.: The World Publishing Company.

Reinhardt, Uwe. 1972. "A Production Function for Physician Services." *Review of Economics and Statistics* 54 (January).

Salkever, David S., and Bice, Thomas W. 1979. *Hospital Certificate-of-Need Controls: Impact on Investment, Cost, and Use.* Washington, DC: American Enterprise Institute for Public Policy Research.

Schwartz, William B.; Newhouse, Joseph P.; Bennett, Bruce W.; Williams, Albert P. 1979. "The Progressive Diffusion of Board-Certified Specialists into Non-Urban Towns." Draft. Santa Monica, CA: The Rand Corporation.

Schweitzer, S. O. 1974. "The Cost Effectiveness of Early Detection of Disease." *Health Services Research* 9 (Spring):22–32.

Sloan, Frank A. 1974. "A Microanalysis of Physicians' Hours of Work." In Mark Perlman, ed., *The Economics of Health and Medical Care: Proceedings of a Conference Held by the International Economic Association at Tokyo.* New York: John Wiley and Sons.

————. 1976. "Physician Fee Inflation: Evidence from the late 1960s." In Richard Rosett, ed., *The Role of Health Insurance in the Health Services Sector.* A Conference of the Universities—National Bureau Committee for Economic Research. New York: National Bureau for Economic Research.

————. 1975. "Physician Supply Behavior in the Short Run." *Industrial and Labor Relations Review* 28 (July).

————, and Steinwald, Bruce. 1978. "Effects of Regulation on Hospital Costs and Input Use." Paper presented at the Annual Meeting of the American Economic Association, 29 August (Chicago, Illinois).

Starr, Paul, et al. 1973. *The Discarded Army: Veterans after Vietnam.* New York: Charterhouse.

Stigler, George. 1974. "Free Riders and Collective Action: An Appendix to Theories of Economic Regulation." *Bell Journal of Economics and Management Science* 5, 2 (Autumn):359—65.

Stockman, David A., and Gramm, W. Philip. 1979. "The Administration's Case for 'Hospital Cost Containment': A Critical Analysis." *THA ● Texas Hospital* 35, 1 (June):25—34.

U.S. Department of Health, Education, and Welfare. 1979. *Fact Sheet: President Carter's National Health Plan Legislation* (12 June). Washington, DC: HEW.

————. 1975. *Physician Visits: Volume and Interval since Last Visit, United States— 1971.* Series 10, No. 97, of *Vital and Health Statistics.* Washington, DC: HEW.

————. 1974. "Provisions of Bills Introduced in the 93rd Congress as of February 1974." *National Health Insurance Proposals* (March). Washington, DC: Social Security Administration, Office of Research and Statistics.

U.S. House of Representatives Committee on Appropriations. 1974. *Department of Defense Appropriations for 1975, Part 6, Medical Operations.* Washington, DC: U.S. Government Printing Office.

U.S. Senate Committee on Finance. 1979. "Presentation of Major Health Insurance Proposals, Hearings, June 19 and 21, 1979." Washington, DC: U.S. Government Printing Office.

Ziderman, A. 1971. "Incremental Rates of Return on Investment in Education: Recent Results for Britain." Mimeo. Queen Mary College, University of London.

ABOUT THE AUTHORS

ALAIN ENTHOVEN is Marriner S. Eccles Professor of Public and Private Management, Stanford Graduate School of Business, and Professor of Health Care Economics in the Department of Family, Community, and Preventive Medicine at the Stanford School of Medicine. His experience in economics and public health care policy includes MIT, The Rand Corporation, The Brookings Institution, and ten years spent in research analysis at the Department of Defense. He has been a member of the Visiting Committee of the Harvard School of Public Health since 1974. His many articles include "Medical Care Costs: Where to Go from Here?" (*National Journal*, 1976), "Consumer-Centered vs. Job-Centered Health Insurance" (*Harvard Business Review*, 1979), and "Consumer-Choice Health Plan: A National Health Insurance Proposal Based on Regulated Competition in the Private Sector" (*New England Journal of Medicine*, 1978).

W. PHILIP GRAMM, U.S. Congressman from the 6th District of Texas, is a former Professor of Economics at Texas A. & M. University. He has been consultant to the U.S. Bureau of Mines, the National Science Foundation, the Arms Control and Disarmament Agency, and the U.S. Public Health Service. He is the author of several books and monographs, including articles published in the *American Economic Review*, the *Journal of Money, Credit and Banking*, and the *Journal of Economic History*, and guest editorials in the *Wall Street Journal* and *National Observer*.

LEON R. KASS is Henry R. Luce Professor in the College, The University of Chicago. He is a former Joseph P. Kennedy, Sr., Research Professor in Bioethics at The Kennedy Institute and Associate Professor of Neurology and of Philosophy at Georgetown University. A member of the American Association for the Advancement of Science and of the Board of Directors of the Institute of Society, Ethics, and the Life Sciences, much of Dr. Kass's writing has dealt with ethical issues in medical practice, including his 1975 article in *The Public Interest* entitled "Regarding the End of Medicine and the Pursuit of Health."

KEITH B. LEFFLER, Assistant Professor of Economics at the University of Washington, shows a keen interest in the economics of health care services. He wrote "National Health Insurance: A Social Placebo?" (*Current History*, 1977), and in 1979 he was the author of a guest editorial in the *Wall Street Journal* entitled "Doctors' Fees and Health Costs."

COTTON M. LINDSAY is Associate Professor of Economics at UCLA and in 1979 became Visiting Professor and Director of the EAGLE Institute in the School of Business Administration at Emory University in Atlanta, Georgia. A former National Fellow at the Hoover Institution, Stanford University, much of his writing has been concerned with medical economics. His books include, in addition to his work on Canadian and British health insurance systems, *Veterans Administration Hospitals: An Economic Analysis of Government Enterprise* (1975), and *The Pharmaceutical Industry: Economics, Performance and Government Regulation* (1978), which he edited. Two forthcoming articles in 1980 will be "Medical Schools: Producers of What? Sellers to Whom?" written with Thomas D. Hall, to appear in *The Journal of Law and Economics*, and, with Keith Leffler, "Markets for Medical Care and Medical Education: An Integrated Long-Run Structural Approach" for *The Journal of Human Resources*.

JACK A. MEYER is Director of the Office of Special Projects at the American Enterprise Institute for Public Policy Research in Washington, DC. His experience as an economist includes the direction of the Office of Special Studies at the Department of Housing and Urban Development, and three years with the president's Council on Wage and Price Stability including the position of assistant director for Wage and Price Monitoring. He is the author of a paper on wage policy published by OECD (Paris), a number of articles published in the *AEI Economist* and the *Review of Economics and Statistics*, and two recent AEI books—*Health Care Cost Increases* and *Real Wage Insurance*.

CHARLES E. PHELPS, Director of the Regulatory Policies and Institutions Program of The Rand Corporation where he is Senior Staff Economist, served as principal investigator in studying the demand for health insurance and medical care under a grant from HEW. He testified before congressional hearings on national health insurance and participated in national and international conferences on health economics. His many writings on the subject include "Expectations and Realities in National Health Insurance," (*Journal of the Catholic Hospital Association* 1977), "Primary Care, Prevention, and National Health Insurance: A Note of Caution," coauthored with R. L. Kane (forthcoming), and the Rand publication written with J.P. Newhouse and M. S. Marquis, *On Having Your Cake and Eating It Too: Econometric Problems in Estimating the Demand for Health Services* (1979).

THOMAS C. SCHELLING, professor of economics at Harvard University since 1958, is Lucius N. Littauer Professor of Political Economy and chairman of the public administration program at the John Fitzgerald Kennedy School of Government. His experience includes time spent with The Rand Corporation and with the Institute for Strategic Studies (London), and he has been consultant to the Department of State and the Department of Defense, among other government posts. His books include *Micromotives and Macrobehavior* (1978), *Nuclear Power: Issues and Choices* (1977), and the most recent, *Thinking Through the Energy Problem* (1979).

HARRY SCHWARTZ, currently Writer in Residence at the Department of Surgery, College of Physicians and Surgeons, Columbia University, is editorial consultant for *Private Practice* magazine and a member of the editorial board of the *New York Times.* Until 1979 Visiting Professor of Medical Economics at Columbia University and Distinguished Professor, State University of New York at New Paltz, he is the author of many articles that have appeared in the *New England Journal of Medicine, Medical Economics,* the *Wall Street Journal,* and other publications. His nineteen books include *The Case for American Medicine.*

ARTHUR SELDON has been Editorial Director of the Institute of Economic Affairs in London since 1960. A graduate of the London School of Economics, he has been an economist in industry, special adviser to a Cabinet Committee on Welfare of the Commonwealth Government of Australia, and a member of the British Medical Association advisory panel on health service financing. He is a contributor to the *Economist,* the *Financial Times, The Times,* and the *Daily Telegraph.* He is coauthor with Ralph Harris of *Pricing or Taxing?* and *Not from Benevolence,* and wrote "Individual Liberty, Public Goods and Representative Democracy" published by the Hayek Festschrift in *ORDO* (1979).

DAVID A. STOCKMAN, U.S. Congressman for Michigan's 4th District, includes in his committee memberships the Interstate and Foreign Commerce Committee, the president's National Commission on Air Quality, the House Administration Committee, and the subcommittees on Energy and Power and on Health and Environment. Chairman of the Republican Economic Policy Task Force, he is also a member of several Republican Party committees including the National Committee's Advisory Committee on Tax Policy Studies. He was named Executive Director of the House Republican Conference Committee in 1972, a position he resigned in 1975 to run for Congress.

LEWIS THOMAS, President and Chief Executive Officer of Memorial Sloan-Kettering Cancer Center and member of the Sloan-Kettering Institute, is Professor of Pathology and Medicine at the Cornell University Medical College, Adjunct Professor at Rockefeller University, and consultant to the Rockefeller University Hospital. He has held government positions on national and New York City advisory and research boards and is currently a member of many national and international committees and advisory groups. His book, *The Lives of a Cell*, won the 1974 National Book Award in Arts and Letters.

INDEX

SELECTED PUBLICATIONS FROM
THE INSTITUTE FOR CONTEMPORARY STUDIES
260 California Street, San Francisco, California 94111
Catalog available upon request

THE CALIFORNIA COASTAL PLAN: A CRITIQUE
$5.95. 199 pages. Publication date: March 1976.
ISBN 0-917616-04-9
Library of Congress No. 76-7715
Contributors: Eugene Bardach, Daniel K. Benjamin, Thomas E. Borcherding, Ross D. Eckert, H. Edward Frech, M. Bruce Johnson, Ronald N. Lafferty, Walter J. Mead, Daniel Orr, Donald M. Pach, Michael R. Peevey.

THE CRISIS IN SOCIAL SECURITY: PROBLEMS AND PROSPECTS
$5.95. 214 pages. Publication date: April 1977; 2d ed., rev., 1978.
ISBN 0-917616-16-2, 0-917616-25-1
Library of Congress No. 77-72542
Contributors: Michael J. Boskin, George F. Break, Rita Ricardo Campbell, Edward Cowan, Martin Feldstein, Milton Friedman, Douglas R. Munro, Donald O. Parsons, Carl V. Patton, Joseph A. Pechman, Sherwin Rosen, W. Kip Viscusi, Richard J. Zeckhauser.

DEFENDING AMERICA: TOWARD A NEW ROLE IN THE POST-DETENTE WORLD
$13.95 (hardbound only). 255 pages. Publication date: April 1977 by Basic Books (New York).
ISBN 0-465-01585-9
Library of Congress No. 76-43479
Contributors: Robert Conquest, Theodore Draper, Gregory Grossman, Walter Z. Laqueur, Edward N. Luttwak, Charles Burton Marshall, Paul H. Nitze, Norman Polmar, Eugene V. Rostow, Leonard Schapiro, James R. Schlesinger, Paul Seabury, W. Scott Thompson, Albert Wohlstetter.

EMERGING COALITIONS IN AMERICAN POLITICS
$6.95. 530 pages. Publication date: June 1978.
ISBN 0-917616-22-7
Library of Congress No. 78-53414

287

Contributors: Jack Bass, David S. Broder, Jerome M. Clubb, Edward H.
Crane III, Walter De Vries, Andrew M. Greeley, Tom Hayden, S. I.
Hayakawa, Milton Himmelfarb, Richard Jensen, Paul Kleppner,
Everett Carll Ladd, Jr., Seymour Martin Lipset, Robert A. Nisbet,
Michael Novak, Gary R. Orren, Nelson W. Polsby, Joseph L. Rauh,
Jr., Stanley Rothman, William A. Rusher, William Schneider, Jesse
M. Unruh, Ben J. Wattenberg.

FEDERAL TAX REFORM: MYTHS AND REALITIES

$5.95. 270 pages. Publication date: September 1978.
ISBN 0-917616-32-4
Library of Congress No. 78-61661

Contributors: Robert J. Barro, Michael J. Boskin, George F. Break, Jerry
R. Green, Laurence J. Kotlikoff, Mordecai Kurz, Peter
Mieszkowski, John B. Shoven, Paul J. Taubman, John Whalley.

GOVERNMENT CREDIT ALLOCATION: WHERE DO WE GO FROM HERE?

$4.95. 208 pages. Publication date: November 1975.
ISBN O-917616-02-2
Library of Congress No. 75-32951

Contributors: George Benston, Karl Brunner, Dwight Jaffe, Omotunde
Johnson, Edward J. Kane, Thomas Mayer, Allen H. Meltzer.

NEW DIRECTIONS IN PUBLIC HEALTH CARE: AN EVALUATION OF PROPOSALS FOR NATIONAL HEALTH INSURANCE

$5.95. 277 pages. Publication date: May 1976.
ISBN 0-917616-06-5
Library of Congress No. 76-9522

Contributors: Martin S. Feldstein, Thomas D. Hall, Leon R. Kass, Keith B.
Leffler, Cotton M. Lindsay, Mark V. Pauly, Charles E. Phelps,
Thomas C. Schelling, Arthur Seldon.

NEW DIRECTIONS IN PUBLIC HEALTH CARE: A PRESCRIPTION FOR THE 1980s

$6.95. 300 pages. Publication date: May 1976; 3d ed. rev., 1980.
ISBN 0-917616-37-5
Library of Congress No. 79-92868

Contributors: Alain Enthoven, W. Philip Gramm, Leon R. Kass, Keith B.
Leffler, Cotton M. Lindsay, Jack A. Meyer, Charles E. Phelps, Thomas
C. Schelling, Harry Schwartz, Arthur Seldon, David A. Stockman, Lewis
Thomas

NO LAND IS AN ISLAND: INDIVIDUAL RIGHTS AND GOVERN-
MENT CONTROL OF LAND USE
$5.95. 221 pages. Publication date: November 1975.
ISBN 0-917616-03-0
Library of Congress No. 75-38415
Contributors: Benjamin F. Bobo, B. Bruce-Briggs, Connie Cheney, A. Law-
rence Chickering, Robert B. Ekelund, Jr., W. Philip Gramm, Donald G.
Hagman, Robert B. Hawkins, Jr., M. Bruce Johnson, Jan Kras-
nowiecki, John McClaughry, Donald M. Pach, Bernard H. Siegan,
Ann Louise Strong, Morris K. Udall.

NO TIME TO CONFUSE: A CRITIQUE OF THE FORD FOUNDA-
TION'S ENERGY POLICY PROJECT *A TIME TO CHOOSE AMERICA'S
ENERGY FUTURE*
$4.95. 156 pages. Publication date: February 1975.
ISBN 0-917616-01-4
Library of Congress No. 75-10230
Contributors: Morris A. Adelman, Armen A. Alchian, James C. DeHaven,
George W. Hilton, M. Bruce Johnson, Herman Kahn, Walter J. Mead,
Arnold B. Moore, Thomas Gale Moore, William H. Riker.

ONCE IS ENOUGH: THE TAXATION OF CORPORATE EQUITY
INCOME
$2.00. 32 pages. Publication date: May 1977.   .
ISBN 0-917616-23-5
Library of Congress No. 77-670132
Author: Charles E. McLure, Jr.

OPTIONS FOR U.S. ENERGY POLICY
$5.95. 317 pages. Publication date: September 1977.
ISBN 0-917616-20-0
Library of Congress No. 77-89094
Contributors: Albert Carnesale, Stanley M. Greenfield, Fred S. Hoffman,
Edward J. Mitchell, William R. Moffat, Richard Nehring, Robert
S. Pindyck, Norman C. Rasmussen, Davis J. Rose, Henry S. Rowen,
James L. Sweeney, Arthur W. Wright.

PARENTS, TEACHERS, AND CHILDREN: PROSPECTS FOR CHOICE
IN AMERICAN EDUCATION
$5.95. 336 pages. Publication date: June 1977.
ISBN 0-917616-18-9
Library of Congress No. 77-79164
Contributors: James S. Coleman, John E. Coons, William H. Cornog,
Denis P. Doyle, E. Babette Edwards, Nathan Glazer, Andrew
M. Greeley, R. Kent Greenawalt, Marvin Lazerson, William
C. McCready, Michael Novak, John P. O'Dwyer, Robert Singleton,
Thomas Sowell, Stephen D. Sugarman, Richard E. Wagner.

THE POLITICS OF PLANNING: A REVIEW AND CRITIQUE OF
CENTRALIZED ECONOMIC PLANNING
$5.95. 352 pages. Publication date: March 1976.
ISBN 0–917616–05–7
Library of Congress No. 76–7714
Contributors: B. Bruce-Briggs, James Buchanan, A. Lawrence Chickering,
Ralph Harris, Robert B. Hawkins, Jr., George Hilton, Richard Man-
cke, Richard Muth, Vincent Ostrom, Svetozar Pejovich, Myron
Sharpe, John Sheahan, Herbert Stein, Gordon Tullock, Ernest van den
Haag, Paul H. Weaver, Murray L. Weidenbaum, Hans Willgerodt,
Peter P. Witonski.

PUBLIC EMPLOYEE UNIONS: A STUDY OF THE CRISIS IN PUBLIC
SECTOR LABOR RELATIONS
$5.95. 251 pages. Publication date: June 1976; 2d ed., rev., 1977.
ISBN 0–917616–08–1, 0–917616–24–3
Library of Congress No. 76–17444
Contributors: A. Lawrence Chickering, Jack D. Douglas, Raymond
D. Horton, Theodore W. Kheel, David Lewin, Seymour Martin
Lipset, Harvey C. Mansfield, Jr., George Meany, Robert A. Nisbet,
Daniel Orr, A. H. Raskin, Wes Uhlman, Harry H. Wellington,
Charles B. Wheeler, Jr., Ralph K. Winter, Jr., Jerry Wurf.

REGULATING BUSINESS: THE SEARCH FOR AN OPTIMUM
$5.95. 300 pages. Publication date: April 1978
ISBN 0–917616–27–8
Library of Congress No. 78–50678
Contributors: Chris Argyris, A. Lawrence Chickering, Penny Hollander
Feldman, Richard H. Holton, Donald P. Jacobs, Alfred E. Kahn,
Paul W. MacAvoy, Almarin Phillips, V. Kerry Smith, Paul H.
Weaver, Richard J. Zeckhauser.

WATER BANKING: HOW TO STOP WASTING
AGRICULTURAL WATER
$2.00. 56 pages. Publication date: January 1978.
ISBN 0–917616–26–X
Library of Congress No. 78–50766
Authors: Sotirios Angelides, Eugene Bardach.